Navigating AI in Mental Health Care

Susmita Halder · Bibhrajit Halder ·
Akash Kumar Mahato

Navigating AI in Mental Health Care

Innovations, Ethics, and Future Trends

Springer

Susmita Halder
Department of Psychology
St. Xavier's University
Kolkata, West Bengal, India

Bibhrajit Halder
SafeAI
Santa Clara, CA, USA

Akash Kumar Mahato
Department of Clinical Psychology
Amity University
Newtown, West Bengal, India

ISBN 978-981-96-9743-4 ISBN 978-981-96-9744-1 (eBook)
https://doi.org/10.1007/978-981-96-9744-1

This Springer imprint is published by the registered company Springer Nature Singapore Pte Ltd.
The registered company address is: 152 Beach Road, #21-01/04 Gateway East, Singapore 189721, Singapore

Preface

Artificial Intelligence (AI) is definitely the biggest thing that has happened to humanity after the internet. AI is the buzzword that has engulfed each and every domain humans engage for occupation, interact and communicate, do business, learn, entertain, or create something with its promising potential. With its growing effectiveness and fine-tuning AI is reshaping the world, by reducing human effort, and improving capacity parallelly in all domains we can think of, including health care. However, there still lies a lot of apprehensions when it comes to the domain of health, particularly mental health, where human interface and communication between a professional and patient are vital for both diagnostic and therapeutic processes. So how does AI fit into this? There is an upward trend of references and books which speak volumes about the promising role of AI in mental health; however, it is important to bring AI experts and mental health experts on the same platform as both are mostly novice about the nuances of each other's field.

Through this book, we try to not only highlight the applications of AI in mental health, but more importantly undertake to highlight major domains in mental health, where specific AI inputs are required. We attempt to highlight or identify 'statements of problem' in major mental ill health conditions where AI can have a specific role.

West Bengal, India — Susmita Halder
Santa Clara, USA — Bibhrajit Halder
West Bengal, India — Akash Kumar Mahato

Acknowledgements The book would not have been possible without valuable inputs and contribution from Shouvik Basak. Would like to thank Shinjini Samajdar for her inputs in the process.

Competing Interests The authors have no competing interests to declare that are relevant to the content of this manuscript.

Contents

About the Authors

Susmita Halder is Accomplished Academician, Researcher, and Clinical Psychologist with more than 20 years of experience in teaching and consultancy. She is currently Professor in Psychology at St. Xavier's University, Kolkata. She has keen interest in studying human behaviour and connecting it with daily life and brain functioning and applying modern psychotherapies to improve one's mental health and wellness. She had been Research Fellow at the prestigious Centre for the Study of Developing Societies, New Delhi. She has worked with leading academic institutions and super specialty hospitals in India. She gainfully uses her experiences into her work and writings. She is the author of the book, "Healthy Brain: Way to Healthy life" and editor of the book "Mental Health in Ageing: Current Perspectives". She also has over 100 research publications and has presented talks and seminars on national and international platforms.

Dr. Bibhrajit Halder is Founder and CEO of SafeAI, Leader in autonomous technology and solutions for heavy vehicles, headquartered at Santa Clara, CA, USA. Dr. Bibhrajit has been involved in the autonomy industry for over 20 years and worked on self-driving projects at Caterpillar, Ford, Faraday Future, and Apple before founding SafeAI in 2017. He holds a Ph.D. in Mechanical Engineering from Vanderbilt University and an M.S. in Mathematics and Mechanical Engineering from Ohio University.

Akash Kumar Mahato is Associate Professor in Clinical Psychology and Head of the Amity Institute of Psychology and Allied Sciences, Amity University, Kolkata. An alumnus of the Ranchi Institute of Neuro-Psychiatry and Allied Sciences; Dr. Mahato has an experience of over 16 years in the industry and academia. Previously, he had been faculty and Principal at Sweekaar Academy of Rehabilitation Sciences, Secunderabad. He has also contributed as faculty and Clinical Psychologist in Postgraduate teaching departments in medical colleges and Universities in the past including LGB Regional Institute of Mental Health, Assam, and Amity University, Jaipur. His interest areas lie in Evidence-based Psychotherapy, Therapeutic indication of Neuro-cognitive functions, and Community Mental Health. Dr. Mahato has over 50 peer-reviewed, national and international publications to his credit.

Abbreviations

AI	Artificial Intelligence
AR	Augmented Reality
CBT	Cognitive-Behavioural Therapy
DL	Deep Learning
Gen AI	Generative AI
LLMs	Large Language Models
ML	Machine Learning
NLP	Natural Language Processing
VR	Virtual Reality
W.H.O	World Health Organisation

Part I
Introduction

Chapter 1
Essentials of Mental Health

Abstract Most of us have a fair perception of conditions like depression and anxiety and consider their presence or absence in our lives as an indicator of good or bad mental health. The concept of mental health, though broadly includes anxiety and depression, is much wider than this. Absence of mental disorders, while desirable, is not the absolute indicator of good mental health, which exists on a complex continuum, is experienced differently by different individuals with varying degrees of difficulty and distress and potentially very different social and clinical outcomes (WHO in Mental health and COVID-19: Early evidence of the pandemic's impact. World Health Organization, 2022). In this chapter, we provide an overview of mental health basics and their everyday relevance. The global prevalence of mental health challenges, and its social, cultural, and economic dimensions and impact is examined. Additionally, we introduce key elements, such as emotional resilience, stress management, and social support. The chapter underscores the importance of early detection and intervention for mental health issues, emphasizing the pivotal role mental well-being plays in individual and societal health.

Keywords Mental health · Disorders · Well-being · Brain · Treatment

Overview

The awareness regarding mental health has grown positively and globally in recent years. More importantly, mental health is not seen as a separate category of health, rather integral component of one's health, as the World Health Organisation (WHO) defines health as "a state of complete physical, mental, and social well-being, not merely the absence of disease or infirmity". This highlights the importance of mental health in overall health. Dr. Margaret Chan, former Director-General of the World Health Organisation, emphasized that good mental health is vital and enables people to realize their potential and cope with normal stresses, in addition to aiding to work productively and contribute to their communities.

S. Halder et al., *Navigating AI in Mental Health Care*,
https://doi.org/10.1007/978-981-96-9744-1_1

Grasping these fundamentals of mental health is essential for nurturing a society that values and prioritizes well-being of its members. Acknowledging the widespread impact of mental health problems worldwide, it is imperative to create a more compassionate and supportive environment. This chapter serves as the cornerstone for further exploration into the multifaceted realm of mental health and advocates for a society that places mental well-being on equal footing with physical health, benefiting all.

Unlike physical health, mental health concerns are often less visible but equally impactful. Historically, mental health was misunderstood and stigmatized; only recently have awareness and advocacy efforts begun to reduce this stigma. Mental health includes aspects of emotional resilience, stress management, and relationships, as well as the absence of mental disorders. Awareness of mental health is increasingly recognized as crucial in public health, particularly in today's fast-paced society where stress-related issues are widespread. Awareness is also vital to remove stigma attached with mental health issues, as stigmatization remains a significant barrier to accessing mental health care, underscoring the importance of awareness and open discussions on mental health issues (WHO, 2021).

Epidemiology of Mental Disorders

Mental disorders affect millions of people each year, globally. According to the World Health Organization, depression is a leading cause of disability worldwide, and anxiety disorders affect around 264 million people. Epidemiology examines patterns in mental health issues, identifying groups most affected by disorders and how factors such as age, gender, and socioeconomic status influence mental health. For example, younger adults and adolescents are more prone to anxiety and mood disorders, while older populations experience increased rates of cognitive decline and depression. Understanding these patterns helps inform public health policies and intervention programmes to address the burden of mental illness in diverse populations (WHO, 2019; NIMH, 2021; CDC, 2020). Mental diseases are known to contribute significantly to long-term incapacity and reliance. Mental diseases significantly increase the global disease burden. The World Health Organization's 2005 global illness burden estimates demonstrate the impact of health issues globally. It mentions non-communicable illnesses fast becoming the leading cause of illness in all emerging regions except Sub-Saharan Africa. The Global Burden of Illness report uses an integrated measure of illness burden, the disability-adjusted life-year, to assess the impact of mental disorders. This measure includes years lived with impairment as well as years lost. As per the report, neuropsychiatric diseases accounted for 31.7 per cent of all years lived with disability. The top five contributors are unipolar depression (11.8%), alcohol use disorder (3.3%), schizophrenia (2.8%), bipolar depression (2.4%), and dementia (1.6%).

The relationship between mental disorders and handicap is more nuanced and comprehensive than the WHO study indicates. While depression is associated with the beginning and progression of physical and social disabilities, disability is a significant risk factor for depression in older persons, mediating the effects of certain physical health disorders. On the other hand, support from society is an effect modifier.

Components of Mental Health

Mental health is crucial at every stage of life, from childhood and adolescence through adulthood. It is a multifaceted aspect of human well-being that encompasses emotional, psychological, and social dimensions. It has been a challenge for researchers and health organizations to have a universal concept of mental health due to cultural differences and they have worked to develop an inclusive definition avoiding limiting assumptions. Majorly, there was no universal agreement on associating mental health with wellness or functioning properly, resulting in a definition that encompasses a wide variety of emotional states and "imperfect functioning". Individuals with positive mental health have described with personality attributes of sense of self competence, and adaptability, who are capable of mastering their environments, as well as identifying, confronting, and solving challenges. Cultural, economic, and political factors all have a significant impact on mental health.

It is important to note that just like physical health, a positive state of mental health requires maintaining healthy behaviours in a continuum and is not a one-day task. Some of the related concepts that contribute to mental health include:

Emotional well-being: It refers to the ability of an individual to understand and manage one's emotions effectively. It involves being aware of one's feelings, expressing them appropriately, and coping with stress in a healthy way. People with good emotional well-being are generally able to maintain a positive outlook on life and navigate through difficult situations with resilience.

Psychological well-being: It encompasses aspects such as self-esteem, resilience, and a sense of purpose in life. It involves having a positive attitude towards oneself and others, feeling competent in one's abilities, and being able to adapt to change and cope with adversity. Psychological well-being is closely linked to mental health, as it influences how individuals perceive and interact with the world around them.

Social well-being refers to the quality of relationships and social support networks that individuals have. It involves feeling connected to others, having a sense of belonging, and being able to build and maintain healthy relationships. Social well-being is essential for mental health, as strong social connections can provide emotional support and help individuals cope with stress.

Mental health is crucial at every stage of life and is the foundation for emotional, psychological, and social well-being throughout the lifespan.

Significance of Mental Health

Here's a deeper dive into why mental health is so crucial: mental health plays a vital role in cognitive functions such as learning, problem-solving, and decision-making. A person's mental well-being directly impacts their ability to concentrate, process information, and retain knowledge. Mental health significantly affects emotional well-being, influencing how individuals experience and express emotions. Good mental health allows for a range of emotions to be experienced and managed appropriately, contributing to resilience in the face of challenges. Mental health influences behaviour, affecting how individuals interact with others and respond to situations. Healthy mental functioning enables individuals to maintain positive relationships, communicate effectively, and engage in productive activities. Good mental health enables individuals to cope and manage stress effectively, preventing it from negatively impacting their physical health and overall well-being.

There is a strong link between mental and physical health. Poor mental health can contribute to the development of physical health problems or aggravation of existing health problems, while good mental health can have a positive impact on physical health and recovery from illness. It allows individuals to adapt to change, learn from experiences, and develop new skills, contributing to personal and professional success.

Brain and Mental Health

The brain is the command centre of the human body, responsible for regulating thoughts, emotions, and behaviours. It contains billions of neurons that communicate through a complex network of synapses, enabling us to respond to stimuli, form memories, and make decisions. When this delicate balance is maintained, we experience good mental health. However, when disruptions occur in the brain's chemistry, structure, or function, they can lead to mental health issues, affecting how we feel, think, and behave.

Mental health disorders, such as depression, anxiety, and schizophrenia, are some of the conditions that arise when the brain's normal processes are altered. While everyone feels sad or anxious from time to time, these feelings usually subside once the stressful situation passes. However, when emotions like sadness or anxiety persist and interfere with daily life, they may indicate the presence of a mental health disorder. Neurotransmitters, the brain's chemical messengers, play a vital role in mental health. For instance, serotonin influences mood and is closely linked to depression; dopamine, involved in reward and pleasure, is associated with disorders like schizophrenia. GABA and norepinephrine are also essential, affecting anxiety and stress responses. When neurotransmitter systems are imbalanced, mood, perception, and behaviour can be impacted, contributing to various mental health conditions. For example, reduced serotonin levels are often associated with depressive symptoms, while dysregulation of dopamine can contribute to schizophrenia and psychotic symptoms. Understanding these mechanisms has led to advancements in psychotropic medications aimed at restoring neurotransmitter balance (Stahl, 2013; Nestler et al., 2019).

From a neuropsychological perspective, mental health is about maintaining a state of balance in our brain's functions, allowing us to navigate life's challenges effectively and find joy and satisfaction in our daily activities. It is important to note that mental illnesses can range in severity, from mild cases that cause minor disruptions to severe forms that can be debilitating.

Mental illnesses are often misunderstood due to various myths and misconceptions. For instance, people might assume that individuals with mental illnesses always exhibit visible symptoms, such as erratic behaviour or emotional instability. However, many mental health disorders can be subtle, especially in their early stages. A person may appear outwardly normal while struggling internally with symptoms like persistent sadness, fatigue, or a sense of hopelessness. Conditions like depression and anxiety often go unnoticed because they do not always manifest in obvious ways, making it crucial to pay attention to changes in mood, behaviour, and overall functioning.

There are different types of mental health disorders, each affecting the brain in distinct ways. Depression, for example, is a common mental illness characterized by prolonged feelings of sadness, loss of interest, and changes in sleep and appetite. It is associated with imbalances in the brain, particularly involving neurotransmitters like serotonin and dopamine, which regulate mood. Schizophrenia, on the other hand, is a severe mental disorder that affects how a person thinks, feels, and perceives reality. People with schizophrenia may experience hallucinations, delusions, and disorganized thinking, which significantly impact their ability to lead a normal life. Attention deficit hyperactivity disorder (ADHD) is another example of a mental health condition, typically seen in children but also affecting adults. It involves issues with focus, impulsivity, and hyperactivity, often disrupting daily activities and academic performance.

It is important to distinguish between mental illnesses and neurological disorders, even though they both affect the brain. Neurological disorders, such as epilepsy, Parkinson's disease, and multiple sclerosis, are caused by structural and functional abnormalities in the brain and nervous system. They are generally categorized as brain disorders rather than mental illnesses. However, recent research suggests that the boundary between neurological and mental disorders is not as clear-cut as once believed. Scientists have found that many mental illnesses, like depression and schizophrenia, also involve changes in brain structure, chemistry, and function, highlighting the biological basis of these conditions.

The evolving understanding of mental illness as a brain-based condition is significant because it challenges outdated notions that mental health disorders are simply "all in the mind". Instead, it recognizes that mental illnesses have a biological foundation, similar to physical diseases like diabetes or hypertension. This perspective helps reduce the stigma surrounding mental health conditions, encouraging more people to seek help without fear of judgement. It also emphasizes the need for research into the brain's role in mental health, as understanding the underlying mechanisms can lead to better treatments and interventions.

Major Mental Ill Health Conditions

Some of the major conditions reported in adult mental health clinics are as follows. The list is not exhaustive and does not include childhood disorders.

Mood Disorders: Mood disorders encompass a range of conditions primarily affecting emotional states, including depression and bipolar disorder. Depression is characterized by persistent sadness, loss of interest, and cognitive changes, whereas bipolar disorder involves cycles of mania and depression. Both disorders are influenced by genetic, environmental, and neurobiological factors, and treatments often involve a combination of medication and psychotherapy. Selective serotonin reuptake inhibitors (SSRIs) and mood stabilizers are common pharmacological treatments, while cognitive-behavioural therapy (CBT) is frequently employed to address maladaptive thought patterns (Malhi & Mann, 2018).

Anxiety Disorders: Anxiety disorders include generalized anxiety disorder (GAD), panic disorder, and specific phobias. These conditions are characterized by excessive fear or anxiety that interferes with daily activities. Biological, psychological, and environmental factors contribute to the development of anxiety disorders. Treatment options include CBT, which focuses on restructuring anxious thoughts, and pharmacological interventions, such as benzodiazepines and SSRIs, which target neurotransmitter systems involved in anxiety regulation. Anxiety disorders are among the most common mental health issues, underscoring the need for effective management strategies (Craske et al., 2017; NIMH, 2021).

Obsessive–Compulsive Disorders: Obsessive–compulsive disorder (OCD) involves unwanted, intrusive thoughts (obsessions) and repetitive behaviours (compulsions) aimed at reducing distress. OCD is highly disabling and often coexists with anxiety or depressive disorders. Treatment includes exposure and response prevention (a type of CBT) and medication such as SSRIs. The efficacy of these treatments reflects the importance of addressing both cognitive and behavioural aspects in managing OCD (Ruscio et al., 2010).

Dissociative Disorders: Dissociative disorders are conditions where a person experiences disruptions or discontinuities in consciousness, identity, memory, and perception. Types include dissociative identity disorder (DID), characterized by the presence of two or more distinct identities, and depersonalization-derealization disorder, where individuals feel detached from themselves or their surroundings. Dissociative amnesia involves memory loss that is not attributable to medical conditions. Aetiology often links these disorders to traumatic experiences, particularly in childhood. Treatment may involve trauma-focused therapies, psychotherapy, and support groups to help individuals integrate fragmented aspects of their identity (Spiegel et al., 2013).

Schizophrenia and Other Psychotic Disorders: Schizophrenia, a severe mental disorder, affects how a person thinks, feels, and behaves, often resulting in hallucinations, delusions, and cognitive challenges. Psychotic symptoms in schizophrenia are thought to result from dopamine dysregulation, among other neurobiological factors. Other psychotic disorders share similar symptoms but vary in duration and intensity. Treatment includes antipsychotic medications to manage symptoms and psychosocial interventions to support functional recovery. Early intervention programmes have demonstrated improved outcomes for those experiencing a first episode of psychosis (Tandon et al., 2012; van Os & Kapur, 2009).

Personality Disorders: Personality disorders are enduring patterns of behaviour, cognition, and inner experience that deviate from cultural norms. These have been conventionally grouped into clusters: Cluster A (odd or eccentric), Cluster B (dramatic or erratic), and Cluster C (anxious or fearful), though the latest versions of the ICD and DSM have shifted from the cluster model. Examples include borderline personality disorder, narcissistic personality disorder, and obsessive–compulsive personality disorder. Personality disorders present diagnostic and treatment challenges due to the persistent nature of the symptoms. Dialectical behaviour therapy (DBT) and cognitive-behavioural approaches are commonly used to address maladaptive patterns (Widiger & Costa, 2012).

Sleep Disorders: Sleep disorders, such as insomnia, hypersomnia, and circadian rhythm disorders, significantly impact an individual's overall health and mental well-being. Chronic sleep problems are linked to mood disorders, anxiety, and impaired cognitive function. Treatments include cognitive-behavioural therapy for insomnia (CBT-I), sleep hygiene education, and, in some cases, medication. Understanding the relationship between sleep and mental health can inform interventions that enhance quality of life (Morin & Benca, 2012).

Sexuality, Gender Dysphoria, and Paraphilias: Gender dysphoria involves distress associated with a mismatch between one's gender identity and assigned sex at birth. Paraphilias include atypical sexual interests, which, when acted upon or causing distress, are termed paraphilic disorders. Treatment may include psychotherapy to support individuals in understanding their identity and managing distress. Ethical considerations are crucial, particularly in providing affirmative care for gender-diverse individuals and ensuring that interventions respect individual rights (Coleman et al., 2012).

Substance-Related Disorders: Substance-related disorders encompass the misuse of alcohol, drugs, and other substances, which can lead to dependency and mental health issues. These disorders often involve compulsive use, tolerance, and withdrawal symptoms, which significantly impact an individual's social and occupational functioning. Treatment includes behavioural therapies, support groups like Narcotics

Anonymous, and medications such as methadone for opioid dependency. Understanding the neurobiological basis of addiction has led to more effective treatments that target cravings and relapse prevention (NIDA, 2020).

Mental Disorders in Special Population Groups

Older Adults and Mental Health Issues: Mental health in older adults presents unique challenges, including depression, anxiety, and cognitive decline. Age-related changes, such as retirement and health deterioration, can increase vulnerability to mental health issues. Barriers to care include stigma, limited mobility, and insufficient social support. Effective interventions involve counselling, community support, and, when appropriate, pharmacological treatment tailored for age-related physiological factors (APA, 2017; WHO, 2017).

Women and Mental Health Issues: Women face unique mental health challenges, including postpartum depression, premenstrual dysphoric disorder (PMDD), and the impact of gender-based violence. Biological factors, such as hormonal fluctuations, and social stressors, like caregiving responsibilities, influence mental health in women. Effective treatment involves acknowledging these unique factors, providing targeted therapies, and fostering support networks (Howard et al., 2014; WHO, 2019).

Children, Adolescents, and Mental Health Issues: Children and adolescents are susceptible to mental health conditions such as attention-deficit/hyperactivity disorder (ADHD), conduct disorders, and mood disorders. Factors like family environment, school stress, and peer relationships significantly affect mental health during these developmental stages. Early diagnosis and intervention, including behavioural therapy and family-based interventions, are essential to support youth mental health and prevent long-term consequences (Kessler et al., 2005; CDC, 2020).

Cultural Factors and Minorities: Cultural beliefs and practices shape mental health perceptions and access to care among ethnic and racial minorities. Minority populations often face higher rates of mental health stigma, language barriers, and systemic discrimination, which impact mental health outcomes and access to resources. Culturally sensitive mental health services and culturally competent therapists are crucial for reducing disparities and enhancing care quality (Gone & Kirmayer, 2010).

The Homelessness Crisis: Mental health issues are prevalent among homeless populations, with higher rates of schizophrenia, bipolar disorder, and substance use disorders compared to the general population. Barriers to accessing mental health care for homeless individuals include lack of resources, stigma, and transient living conditions. Integrated care models, which combine housing, healthcare, and social services, have shown effectiveness in addressing the complex needs of this population (Fazel et al., 2014; Hwang et al., 2019).

Suicides and Homicides: Suicidal and homicidal behaviours are significant concerns within mental health, often linked to mood disorders, substance abuse, and trauma. Risk factors include prior suicide attempts, family history of mental illness, and social isolation. Preventive interventions focus on crisis intervention, suicide hotlines, community support, and public health campaigns aimed at reducing stigma and promoting mental health care (WHO, 2014; Nock et al., 2008).

Improving Mental Health

Taking care of our mental health is as important as taking care of our physical health. Mental health can be influenced by a variety of factors, including genetics, life experiences, trauma, and stress. While some risk factors, such as a family history of mental illness, cannot be changed, others can be managed through healthy lifestyle choices. Regular exercise, a balanced diet, good sleep hygiene, and strong social connections are all vital components of maintaining good mental health. Additionally, developing coping skills, practising mindfulness, and seeking professional help when needed can significantly improve mental well-being. Mental health is a complex and multifaceted aspect of our lives, deeply intertwined with the brain's functions. Understanding the biological basis of mental health disorders helps us appreciate the importance of brain health and reduces the stigma that often surrounds mental illness. By prioritizing mental health and addressing issues early, we can foster a healthier, more resilient society where individuals feel empowered to seek help and support when needed.

Several key components are crucial for ensuring mental health and well-being.

1. The ability to recognize, understand, and manage emotions is essential for mental health. Individuals who can regulate their emotions effectively are better equipped to cope with stress, maintain positive relationships, and make sound decisions.
2. Self-awareness involves understanding one's thoughts, feelings, and behaviours. It allows individuals to recognize when they are experiencing mental health challenges and seek help when needed. Self-awareness also enables individuals to identify their strengths and weaknesses, which can aid in personal growth and development.
3. Strong social connections are vital for mental health. Having supportive relationships can provide comfort, encouragement, and a sense of belonging. Social support can help individuals cope with stress and adversity, reducing the risk of developing mental health problems.
4. A healthy lifestyle that includes regular physical activity, balanced nutrition, adequate sleep, and avoidance of harmful substances is essential for mental health. These lifestyle factors can improve mood, reduce stress, and enhance overall well-being.
5. Effective stress management is crucial for maintaining mental health. Strategies such as mindfulness, relaxation techniques, and time management can help

individuals cope with stressors and prevent the development of mental health problems.

6. Seeking professional help when needed is essential for maintaining mental health. Mental health professionals, such as therapists, counsellors, and psychiatrists, can provide guidance, support, and treatment for a wide range of mental health issues.

By prioritizing emotional regulation, self-awareness, social support, healthy lifestyle habits, stress management, and seeking professional help when needed, individuals can enhance their mental health and lead fulfilling lives. Mental health is closely tied to life satisfaction and investing in mental health can lead to a healthier, happier, and more fulfilling life.

Culture and Mental Health

Each culture influences how individuals see and understand mental health. Ethnic and racial background, as well as genetic factors, influence psychological well-being and mental health in complex ways. Social variables associated with race and ethnicity can lead to inequities in availability of psychological care and resources, affecting mental well-being. While genetics might determine vulnerability to particular situations, interactions with the environment and past experiences are also important. For example, different cultures have different acceptance towards indulgence in taking alcohol, which could be a factor in an individual's propensity to develop alcohol related issues, but at the same time it is also true that people having issue with alcohol are also alarming in countries which taboo alcohol.

The concept of "social capital" has been crucial to the recent resurgence of discussion regarding interpersonal relationships and health promotion. According to Putnam (1995), social capital "refers to features of social organization that include relationships, standards, and trust among individuals that promote interaction and collaboration for mutual benefit". A greater social capital has potential to shield people from social isolation, provide sense of security, improve societal functioning, and boost work performance. In contrary to consolidated individual health outcomes, this view of networks of people who engage with their surroundings has the potential to explain a broader range of collective results.

Perspectives in Treatment of Mental Illnesses

Even though Hippocrates proposed in around 400 BC, that mental illnesses were biological phenomena rather than supernatural, the approach towards treatment or management of mental illness took centuries to appear scientific. Advancements in both pharmacological and non-pharmacological treatment paced in the nineteenth century, and attempts were made globally to shift from custodial treatment and a biological model to biopsychosocial model.

There has been tremendous advancement in development of psychotropic drugs since the 1950s and so, has been the increase in the evidence base of psychotherapeutic managements. While a combination of pharmacological and evidence-based psychotherapies is widely sought after approach, for non-psychotic mental ill health conditions like depression and anxiety spectrum disorders, psychotherapy could be the first choice of treatment, depending on the severity of the symptoms. While psychotropic drugs have refined in terms of their effectiveness, so has the psychotherapeutic approaches which have been customized globally to suit individual clients' socio-cultural background. However, irrespective of what literature or evidence base suggests, the therapeutic requirement of each individual remains unique, and it is gradually becoming evident that the individual seeking therapy is not a passive entity in the process; rather a well-informed client can help moulding the components and process of the therapy and improve treatment outcome. Treatment of individuals with mental illness thus involves pharmacological as well as non-pharmacological interventions, and mostly requires a team or coordinated effort of professionals including psychiatrists, clinical psychologists, and other rehabilitation professionals.

Challenges in Mental Health Care

One of the major challenges that has always plagued delivery of mental health services is disproportionate resources in terms of lesser number of trained professionals, as well as access to mental health services for people from disadvantageous background. The lack of trained professionals is more profound in developing and underdeveloped nations, which puts demanding pressure of existing professionals at all levels, potentially impacting the quality of delivery of the services. The high demand for services often results in long waiting times, and many individuals may not receive the necessary treatment when they need it most.

Even though mental health treatment requires a team effort, there are very few centres which provide all services under one roof, making the process costly and disabling not only for the individual but family at large. In the age of globalization and rapidly changing socio-cultural milieu, less severe but equally disabling mental ill health conditions have increased manifold. The global surge in reported mental health issues post-COVID-19 highlights the need of addressing mental health in all population across all ages. The quality of mental healthcare measures lag behind those developed for physical health, revealing significant gaps in the system's capacity to ensure accountability and drive improvements. Despite ongoing efforts across various organizations, mental health quality indicators remain underdeveloped and inconsistently validated. Although some measures exist, they are not widely implemented or standardized, and their limited scope often emphasizes specific clinical activities or diagnoses without fostering broader systemic changes or enhancing coordination of care. For instance, of the nearly 600 measures endorsed by the National Quality

Forum (NQF), only 16 address mental health issues, demonstrating the limited focus on this critical area of health care. Similarly, in the United States, HEDIS measures only include a fraction dedicated to mental health, underscoring the challenge of promoting comprehensive quality improvement activities within this field.

One of the fundamental challenges in advancing mental health quality measures is the lack of sufficient evidence about what constitutes appropriate care for various conditions. Unlike general health care, where there is a more extensive foundation of evidence-based guidelines, mental health care often lacks robust, conclusive research to inform practice, particularly for certain populations and conditions. For example, there is limited evidence on the appropriate use of atypical antipsychotics in adolescents or the effectiveness of combining antipsychotic medications in adult treatment. Similarly, guidelines for treating bipolar spectrum disorders with antidepressants remain inconclusive, as does the evidence for medication treatment for conditions like PTSD. This gap in evidence poses a significant barrier to developing effective quality measures, as it leaves mental health professionals with few standardized benchmarks against which to assess care quality. Another major issue is the poorly defined parameters that are used to measure mental health care quality. Many key aspects of treatment, such as engagement, psychotherapy, recovery, or intervention fidelity, lack clear and consistent definitions, making it difficult to develop reliable and valid indicators. Furthermore, existing data sources often fall short in providing the necessary information to accurately calculate these indicators. For instance, relying on old ICD-9 codes for mental health diagnoses can be problematic, as these codes may not capture the full complexity of a patient's condition.

Additionally, many quality measures employ strict exclusion criteria that do not reflect the reality of most patients at risk, such as indicators that only consider individuals with newly diagnosed depression. The limited descriptions of mental health care provided by current data sources further hinder their clinical utility, as appropriate pharmacotherapy and psychotherapy data are often scattered across different records, including billing claims and outpatient or pharmacy data. The variability in diagnostic coding practices across mental health services further complicates the interpretation of this data, making it difficult to draw accurate conclusions about the quality of care provided.

Another significant barrier to advancing mental health quality measures is the lack of comprehensive electronic health information systems. In a recent study, only 12% of US hospitals were found to have implemented electronic medical records (EMRs), highlighting the slow adoption of digital record-keeping in the mental health sector. This percentage could be much lower or negligible in developing countries.

Beyond issues of data and measurement, the broader landscape of mental health care faces numerous systemic challenges. Stigma remains a significant barrier, discouraging individuals from seeking help and reducing their engagement with mental health services. The persistent stigma surrounding mental illness contributes to delays in diagnosis and treatment, exacerbating the severity of symptoms and leading to poorer health outcomes.

The variability in insurance coverage for mental health services also complicates access to care. While some policies provide comprehensive coverage, others may have limited benefits or impose strict limits on the number of sessions covered, leaving patients to pay out of pocket. This financial burden can deter individuals from continuing treatment, even when it is clearly needed. Furthermore, the integration of mental health services with primary care remains limited, despite growing recognition of the importance of addressing mental health in conjunction with physical health. Poor coordination between providers can result in fragmented care, where mental health needs are either overlooked or inadequately addressed within the broader health care system. Another significant challenge lies in the development of interventions that are culturally sensitive and tailored to diverse populations. Mental health needs can vary significantly based on cultural, social, and economic factors, and interventions that are effective in one context may not necessarily be suitable in another. The lack of culturally adapted treatment options can lead to disparities in care, as certain groups may not receive interventions that are aligned with their unique needs and preferences. Overall, the field of mental health care faces a multitude of interconnected challenges that hinder the development of effective quality measures and the provision of consistent, high-quality care. Addressing these issues will require coordinated efforts to build a stronger evidence base, enhance data collection systems, and promote greater integration of mental health services across different care settings. By focusing on these areas, it is possible to improve the accountability and quality of mental health care, ultimately leading to better outcomes for individuals suffering from mental health disorders.

The Future with AI Technology

Technology has transformed the landscape of mental health care, creating new avenues for treatment, support, and data collection. The rise of mobile devices like smartphones and tablets has introduced innovative ways for individuals to access mental health services, monitor their progress, and gain insights into their mental well-being. With the growing demand for accessible mental health care, the digital space has become a new frontier, offering a wide range of apps, virtual reality (VR) programmes, and artificial intelligence (AI)-based treatment plans. AI lies at the heart of these advances. The demand of more trained professionals cannot be met overnight, thus, one of the best options seems to divert tasks to assistants who can effectively do the task, and AI seems to be a very eligible assistant at this juncture. Artificial intelligence (AI) has the potential to revolutionize mental health care by enhancing the speed, accuracy, and accessibility of services. AI technologies, such as machine learning and natural language processing, can analyse vast amounts of data to identify patterns and make predictions, aiding in early diagnosis and personalized treatment plans. AI can improve mental health care in several ways, including:

a. AI algorithms can analyse behavioural patterns and identify signs of mental health disorders, enabling early intervention and treatment.

b. AI can analyse individual factors, such as genetics, lifestyle, and environment, to create customized treatment plans that are more effective and tailored to the individual's needs.
c. AI-powered tools, such as chatbots and mobile apps, can provide mental health support and resources to individuals who may not have access to traditional mental health services.
d. AI can accelerate the development of new treatments and interventions by analysing data from clinical trials and research studies.

These advancements are changing how we approach mental health, offering both promising opportunities and notable challenges. Mobile technology has made mental health care more accessible than ever before. Anyone with a phone or computer can now reach out for support through services like the 988 Suicide and Crisis Lifeline, which offers immediate help via call, text, or chat. Beyond these simple yet effective measures, sophisticated apps have emerged, utilizing the built-in sensors of smartphones to track user behaviour patterns. These apps can detect changes in activities such as sleep, movement, or phone usage, which may indicate a potential mental health crisis, prompting timely intervention. Many mental health apps are designed as stand-alone programmes that focus on improving cognitive skills, such as memory or problem-solving. Others facilitate connections with peer counsellors or healthcare professionals, bridging the gap for individuals who might struggle to access traditional in-person therapy. The surge in mobile mental health support has been driven by the need for convenient, cost-effective, and readily accessible treatment options, especially in remote or underserved areas.

Beyond simple communication, more advanced mental health apps are utilizing the sophisticated capabilities of smartphones. Some apps are designed with built-in sensors that can track users' behaviour patterns, such as their movement, sleep, or phone usage. By analysing these data points, the apps can detect deviations from typical behaviour, which may indicate emerging mental health issues. This kind of monitoring allows for early intervention, often before a problem escalates to a crisis level. Other apps focus on enhancing cognitive skills, offering exercises to improve memory or attention, or providing mindfulness and relaxation techniques to help manage stress and anxiety. In some cases, apps also act as a bridge, connecting users directly to mental health professionals or peer counsellors, making the path to receiving help much easier.

The potential benefits of integrating technology into mental health care are vast. One of the primary advantages is convenience; digital tools allow for treatment to be accessed at any time, whether at home during late hours or while commuting. This flexibility is especially beneficial for individuals who have difficulty attending in-person sessions due to time constraints or physical limitations. Additionally, mobile apps offer a level of anonymity that can reduce the stigma often associated with seeking mental health support, encouraging more people to reach out for help without fear of judgement. Cost is another factor that makes digital tools appealing, as many mental health apps are available at low or no cost, making treatment more accessible to a broader audience. For individuals living in remote areas or places with limited mental health resources, these apps can extend the reach of mental health services, providing support that would otherwise be difficult to access. Despite the excitement around mobile mental health technology, there are significant challenges and concerns that need to be addressed. One of the primary issues is the effectiveness of these apps. While thousands of mental health apps are available on platforms like iTunes and the Google Play Store, there is limited scientific evidence to support the effectiveness of many of these tools. This lack of regulation and standardized evaluation makes it difficult for users and healthcare providers to determine which apps are trustworthy and truly beneficial. Privacy is another critical concern, as many mental health apps handle sensitive personal data. Ensuring that this data is protected and not misused is crucial to maintaining user trust and safety.

As more research and engineering teams collaborate, the scope of these apps continues to expand, offering users a wide range of resources to support their mental health. However, with this rapid growth comes the challenge of regulation. Currently, there is no universal standard for evaluating the quality and efficacy of mental health apps, leaving users uncertain about which tools to trust. Overselling the capabilities of these apps come with their unique challenges, as it may give users false confidence or deter them from seeking more effective, traditional therapies when needed, but the future looks promising.

References

Coleman et al. (2012). Standards of Care for the Health of Transsexual, Transgender, and Gender-Nonconforming People, Version 7. *International Journal of Transgenderism, 13*(4), 165–232

Craske, M. G., Stein, M. B., Eley, T. C., Milad, M. R., Holmes, A., Rapee, R. M., & Wittchen, H. U. (2017). Anxiety disorders. Nature reviews. *Disease primers, 3*, 17024.

Howard, L. M., Molyneaux, E., Dennis, C. L., Rochat, T., Stein, A., & Milgrom, J. (2014). Nonpsychotic mental disorders in the perinatal period. *Lancet* (London, England), *384*(9956), 1775–1788.

Kessler, R. C., Berglund, P., Demler, O., Jin, R., Merikangas, K. R., & Walters, E. E. (2005). Lifetime prevalence and age-of-onset distributions of DSM-IV disorders in the National Comorbidity Survey Replication. *Archives of general psychiatry, 62*(6), 593–602.

Malhi, G. S., & Mann, J. J. (2018). Depression. *The Lancet, 392*(10161), 2299–2312.

Morin, C. M., & Benca, R. (2012). Chronic insomnia. *Lancet* (London, England), *379*(9821), 1129–1141.

NIDA (2020). July 6. Drugs and the Brain. Retrieved August 13, 2025, from https://nida.nih.gov/publications/drugsbrains-behavior-science-addiction/drugs-brain

NIMH. (2021). National Institute of Mental Health. (n.d.). Mental illness. U.S. Department of Health and Human Services, National Institutes of Health. Retrieved August 15, 2025, from https://www.nimh.nih.gov/health/statistics/mental-illness

Nestler et al. (2019). The molecular basis of drug addiction: Linking epigenetic to synaptic and circuit mechanisms. *Neuron, 102*(1), 48–59.

Ruscio et al. (2010). The epidemiology of obsessive-compulsive disorder in the National Comorbidity Survey Replication. *Molecular psychiatry, 15*(1), 53–63.

Stahl, S. M. (2013). Classifying psychotropic drugs by mode of action and not by target disorder. *CNS Spectrums, 18*(3), 113–117.

Tandon et al. (2012). Attenuated psychosis and the schizophrenia prodrome: current status of risk identification and psychosis prevention. *Neuropsychiatry, 2*(4), 345–353.
van Os, J., & Kapur, S. (2009). Schizophrenia. *Lancet* (London, England), *374*(9690), 635–645.
Widiger, T. A., & Costa, P. T., Jr (2012). Integrating normal and abnormal personality structure: the Five-Factor Model. *Journal of personality, 80*(6), 1471–1506.
World Health Organization. (2021). *Mental health atlas 2020.* World Health Organization.
World Health Organization. (2022). *Mental health and COVID-19: Early evidence of the pandemic's impact.* World Health Organization.

Chapter 2
Fundamentals of AI

Abstract Artificial intelligence (AI) is definitely one of the most important innovations after the internet. In recent years, AI has emerged as an integral part of our lives and changing the way we live and work, creating value in every domain of our lives. With its inherent ability to follow human instructions (read algorithm) and efficiently perform tasks that would need significant human time and effort, AI has revolutionized numerous sectors, from health care to finance, and its impact continues to grow as the technology advances. The present chapter provides basic understanding of AI and its building blocks, making it easier for readers from different backgrounds to understand the frequently used terminologies in this book.

Keyword Technology · AI · Deep learning · Big data · Mental health care

A Bit of History and Present

Alan Turing, the famous mathematician and computer scientist, introduced the concept of a "universal machine", in 1936, laying the groundwork for modern computing. After fourteen years of this, he proposed the Turing Test to assess a machine's ability to exhibit intelligent behaviour indistinguishable from a human. AI was founded as an academic discipline in the year 1956 at the Dartmouth Conference, where researchers like John McCarthy, Marvin Minsky, Allen Newell, and Herbert Simon introduced the term *artificial intelligence* and set its foundational goals. While the field struggled in its initial years for funding, it grew in prominence from the year 2012, after deep learning was introduced. Global AI funding since 2020 is estimated to be in the range of $300–350 billion.

Perception of common people of AI: All technologies come with baggage of apprehensions. When computers were introduced, people feared it would take their jobs. AI too comes with similar apprehensions but is expected to resolve as it happened with computers. According to the Artificial Intelligence Index Report 2023 (Maslej et al., 2023), people from different countries differ in their opinion about AI being beneficial or having more drawbacks; however, the acceptance regarding AI has grown gradually.

S. Halder et al., *Navigating AI in Mental Health Care*,
https://doi.org/10.1007/978-981-96-9744-1_2

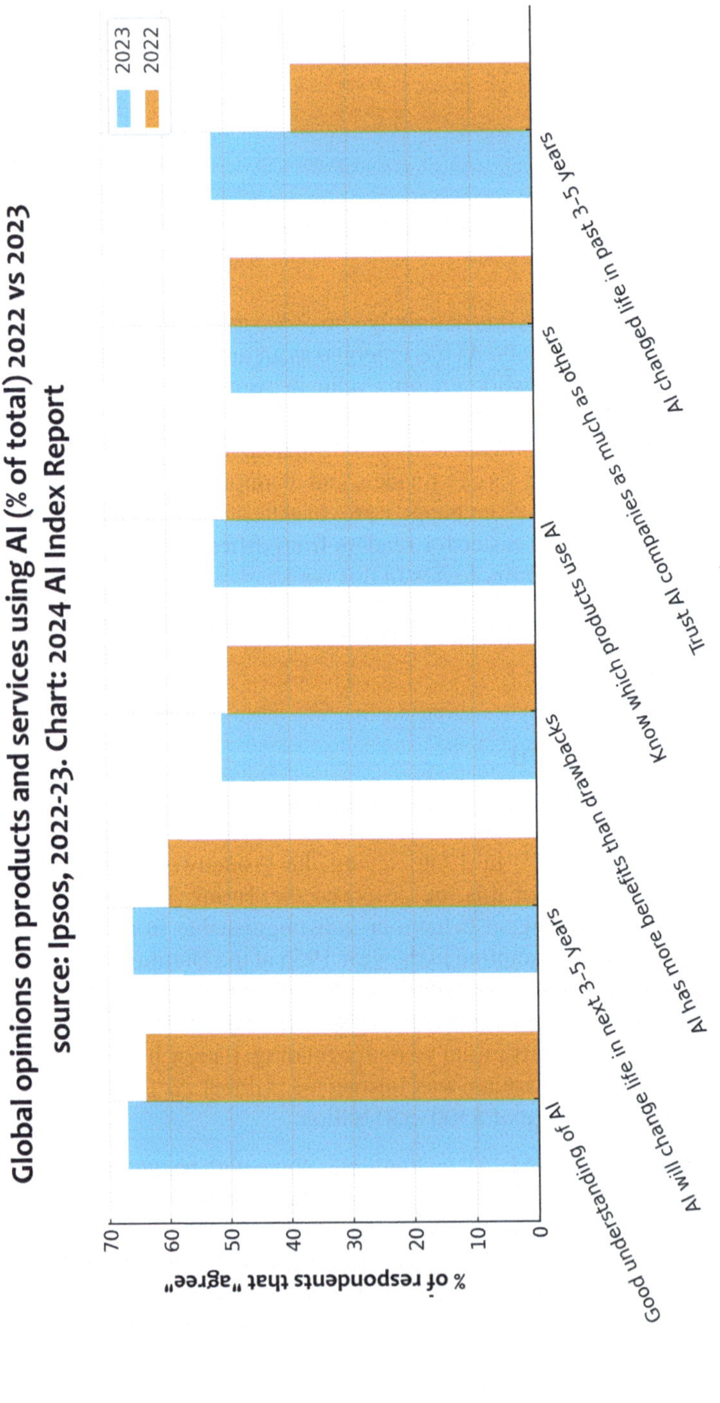

Fig. 2.1 Global Opinions on Products and Services Using AI, comparison of year 2022 vs 2023

Some people worry that AI might take away jobs, but that is not true. In fact, the demand for AI-related professional skills is increasing across industries, and if we learn about AI and adopt it in our practice, we would be able to do our jobs more efficiently. The Artificial Intelligence Index Report 2023 highlights the percentage of all job postings that require some kind of AI skill. For every country included in the sample, AI-related job postings are growing (Figs. 2.1, 2.2).

To be relevant in any industry, it is becoming increasingly necessary to understand AI and be able to adopt and use the tools and techniques embedded with AI in that domain. It is important to acknowledge the disruption coming our way and prepare for the future. We need to be ready for these changes, learn new skills, and adopt AI in our work areas. To be relevant in the industries with the progress happening with AI, we need to know how to leverage AI and get the best out of AI capabilities embedded in various applications.

AI presents tremendous opportunities. Its automation and creative capability can lead to substantial productivity and efficiency gains. However, it comes with its own risks and challenges. One should be aware of these risks, which include unreliability, unpredictability, ethical, and legal concerns. It is crucial to adopt AI to meet the objectives. However, it must be done with caution, being aware of the limitations and risks, and applying the guardrails to prevent potential issues.

Why Do We Need to Know More About AI?

AI technologies are revolutionizing how tasks are performed, reducing time and effort compared to traditional methods. By analysing vast datasets, AI enhances decision-making, uncovers insights, and supports predictive analytics, such as forecasting stock trends or diagnosing diseases. It optimizes processes by automating repetitive tasks, allowing people to focus on creative work. For example, AI can transcribe meetings, summarize discussions, and generate action items, streamlining workflows. Industries are heavily investing in AI, driving cost savings and boosting productivity, while research collaborations between academia and businesses fuel rapid advancements. AI's growing accessibility empowers startups and small businesses to compete with larger organizations, creating opportunities across sectors. As AI integrates into daily life and work, ethical use and responsible development remain key to ensuring its benefits are maximized for all.

AI in Mental Health Care

According to the Artificial Intelligence Index Report (Maslej et al., 2023), in 2022, the AI focus area with the most investment was medical and health care ($6.1 billion); followed by data management, processing, and cloud ($5.9 billion); and Fintech ($5.5 billion). AI is transforming the healthcare domain, including the mental healthcare

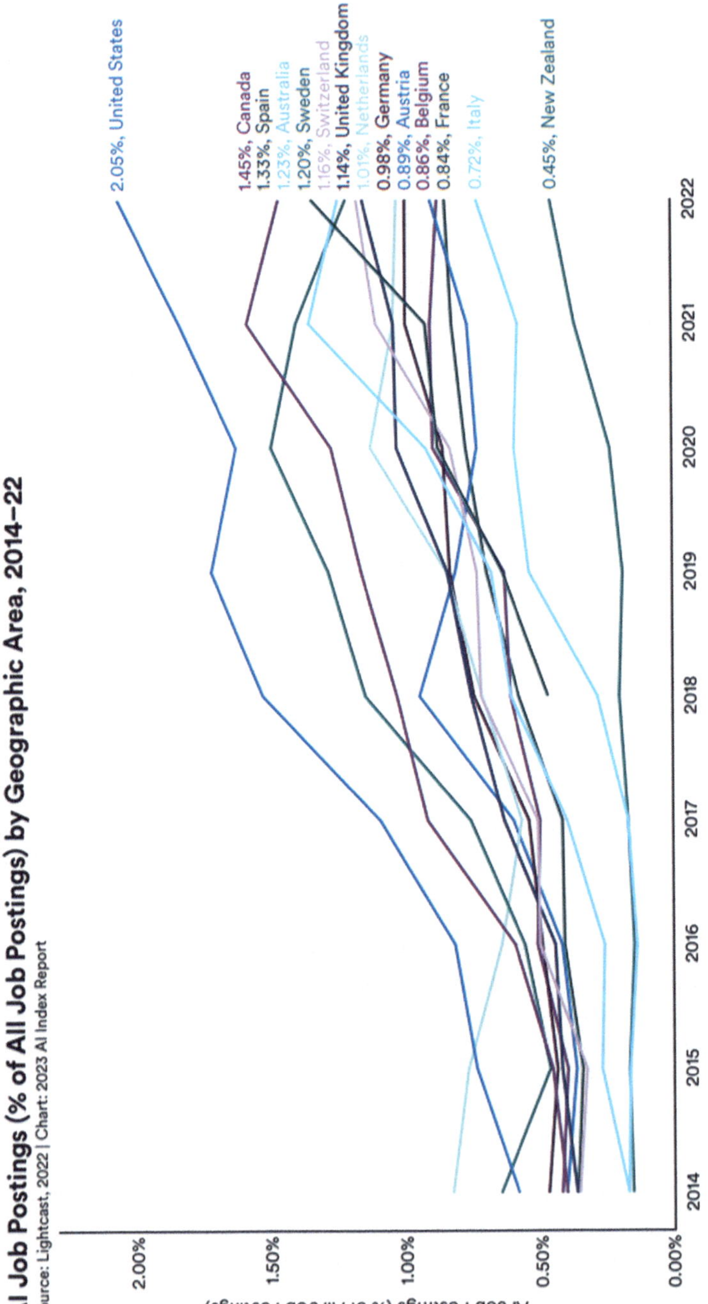

Fig. 2.2 AI Job Postings by Geographic Area- reference

domain. AI is being applied to mental health care for screening, diagnosis, and prognosis. AI applications for mental health care are constantly evolving and are becoming not only an aid for mental health professionals, but for general people to use as a first level support system.

The Fundamental Concepts

AI is helping to build solutions which were once only seen in sci-fi movies and restricted to the development in labs by researchers. Today, it is helping to advance every field whether it be health care, travel, retail, or education. AI is at the core of all the software and applications that are driving the development with incredible capabilities. Let us review the foundations on which these AI capabilities are built.

This chapter introduces the fundamental concepts of AI. It is not meant to teach AI to students interested in building technical solutions or for an aspiring data scientist, but rather to build an awareness of the application of AI for mental health professionals not having a software development and information technology background. It explores the fundamentals of AI and types of solutions that are being built using AI. These are the foundations of the applied tools and techniques used in healthcare services and products, mental health apps, and chatbots. The following sections are the building blocks of various methods and techniques that are discussed in the later chapters of this book.

Machine Learning (ML)

Machine Learning (ML) is the backbone of AI, relying on models built using mathematical and statistical techniques. These models, created as software programmes, learn tasks by analysing large datasets instead of following explicit programming. Through iterative learning, ML models identify patterns, analyse relationships, and make predictions on unseen data.

For example, a retail store with years of sales data, including product details, locations, and buyer demographics, can use ML models to predict future sales trends, identify popular products, and optimize inventory. The data attributes (features) and individual records (samples) feed into the models, which process them using statistical methods to produce outputs (labels). By handling vast datasets, ML models uncover insights and correlations beyond human capacity, enabling accurate predictions and data-driven decision-making. The output that we expect a model to deliver is called a *label*. There may be X number of attributes for each sample and the output is the y, as depicted in Fig. 2.3. So, when an unseen data is passed to a model, all the attributes, $X = \{x_1, x_2, x_3, \ldots x_{10}\}$ is passed as an input to the model for the samples, and y is the output from the model, where the model processes the data based on a mathematical function, f(x).

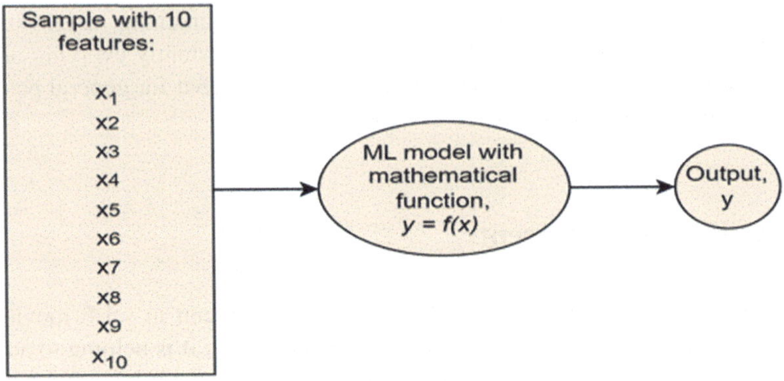

Fig. 2.3 Machine Learning Model

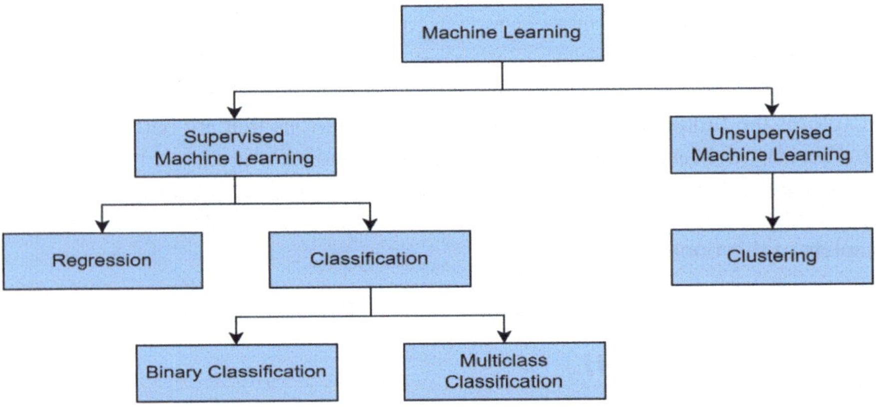

Fig. 2.4 Types of Machine Learning Models

Machine learning models are trained on vast amounts of data to make predictions and draw inferences from the relationships in the data. There are multiple types of machine learning models based on different mathematical techniques and are used for different requirements. Figure 2.4 provides a schematic view of the different types of machine learning models.

Supervised Machine Learning

Supervised machine learning is used when the training data has both *features* and *labels*. The machine learning models are trained on the dataset to learn and determine the relationship between the *features* and *labels*. Broadly there are two types of supervised machine learning models, *regression,* and *classification.*

Regression

Regression is used in cases where the output or *label* is a numeric value determined by a mathematical function, based on the relationship it determines from the features in the *dataset.* Let us understand this by an example. There is a dataset of houses in a city which lists the *features* of the houses, like number of bedrooms, number of bathrooms, number of floors, size of the house in square feet, size of garage, location, and the *label* provided is the price of the house. The machine learning model learns from the relationship of the features and price labels. Based on this learning it builds a model. When an unseen sample with these features is provided as an input to the model, the model predicts the estimated price of the house. The better the model, the model will be able to estimate the potential price more accurately.

Classification

Classification is used where the output label is of a discrete type. For example, given a dataset of features containing various parameters from patient's blood tests, the model may predict whether a patient is diabetic or not. The model classifies two outcomes, diabetic or not diabetic, based on the *label* having the higher probability. These types of classification models are also called *binary classification models* as there can be only two outcomes.

Another type of classification model is *multiclass classification model* where the output can be more than two. For example, a model may take as an input various parameter of flowers and predict whether that flower is a Rose, Sunflower, Tulip, Lily, or Daisy, which are provided as *labels.* As the model determines an output based on multiple outputs, it is called *multiclass* classification models. There is also an extended case for multiclass classification, where the model may be trained for classifying the same sample having more than one output *label.* For example, given a dataset of movie features, the model can classify a movie as romantic and comedy, each being distinct labels.

Unsupervised Machine Learning

Unsupervised machine learning is used when the training data has *features,* but *no labels.* One of the most popular techniques used for unsupervised machine learning is *Clustering.*

Clustering

A clustering algorithm determines the similarities between the features of the various samples, and groups them into discrete clusters. For example, given the photos of cats, dogs, and horses, without providing the model with the labels for the images,

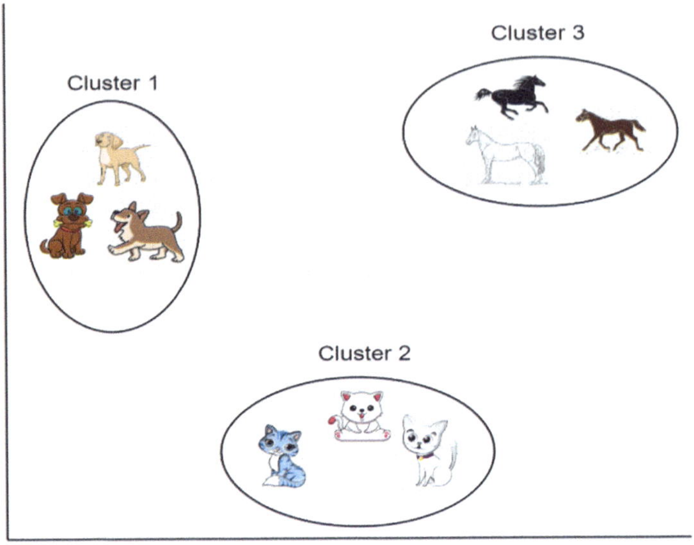

Fig. 2.5 Clustering-reference of figure

the clustering algorithm will group the cats, dogs and horses based on the similarity of the features (Fig. 2.5).

Deep Learning (DL)

On the foundations of machine learning, researchers developed Deep Learning, inspired by how the human brain functions. However, there is no real connection between how the brain functions and how neural networks work. The terms *Deep Learning, Deep Neural Network,* and *Neural Network* are terms often used interchangeably, and they mean the same thing. Deep learning, a subset of machine learning, is a mathematical framework for learning representations from data to perform complex tasks (Fig. 2.6).

The human brain has numerous neurons which fire in response to electromechanical stimuli. Similarly, Neural Networks consist of many *neurons*, which are mathematical functions, that fire based on the input. Artificial Neural Networks are made up of multiple layers of neurons, and hence called the Deep Neural Networks. This led to the term Deep Learning. Deep Learning models or Deep Neural Networks are used for various tasks, including classification, regression, Natural Language Processing (NLP), and Computer Vision.

As an example, deep learning models have been used in medical applications to detect cancer. The deep learning models analyse the images just like medical practitioners would do, however at a massive scale. This kind of analysis may take

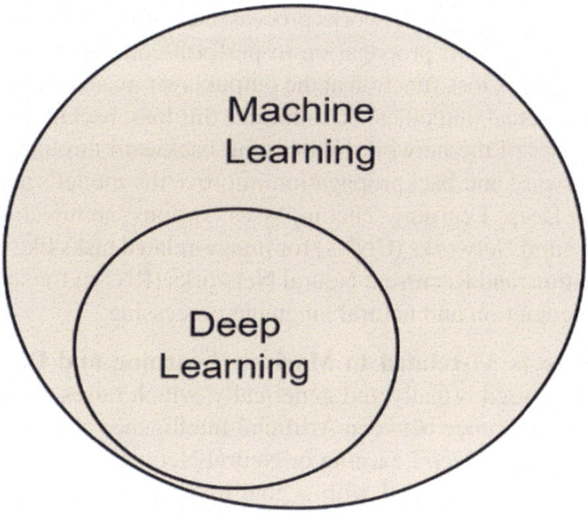

Fig. 2.6 Deep Learning is a subset of Machine Learning

several hours and significant efforts for medical practitioners, but it is done in minutes by these software applications. Researchers have developed AI applications that are making cancer imaging faster, more accurate, and even more informative (Jaber, 2022).

Figure 2.7 shows the schematic of a Neural Network. Let us try to understand how Neural Networks work in a simplified way.

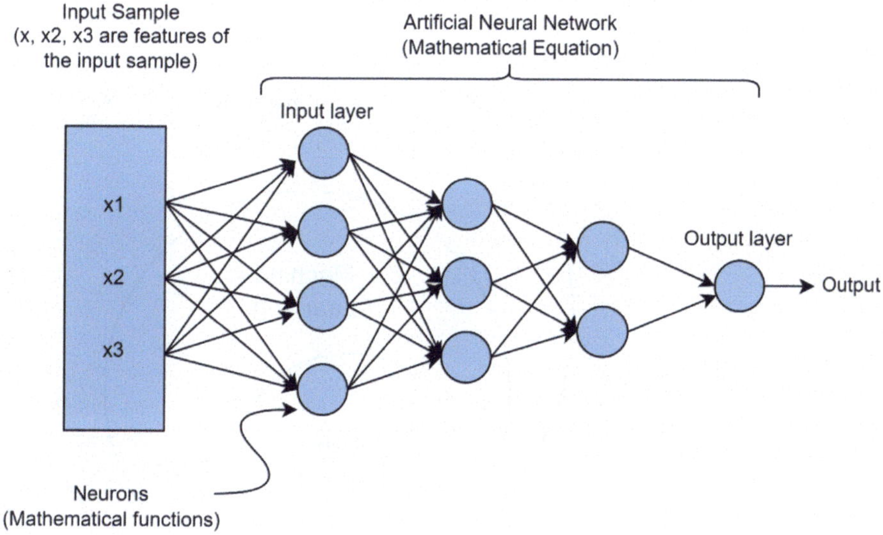

Fig. 2.7 Neural Network

Deep Neural Networks process data through layers of neurons to make predictions, using forward propagation to perform computations at each layer and generate an output. A loss function at the output layer measures the difference between predicted and actual outcomes. To minimize this loss, backpropagation adjusts the weights and biases of the network by iterating backward through the layers. Repeated cycles of forward and backpropagation improve the model's accuracy over time.

Deep Learning encompasses various architectures, including Convolutional Neural Networks (CNNs) for image-related tasks like classification and facial recognition, and Recurrent Neural Networks (RNNs) for sequential data tasks like speech recognition and natural language processing.

How is AI-related to Machine Learning and Deep Learning? Often the term AI is used broadly and generically, which raises the question about what exactly is the difference between Artificial Intelligence and Machine Learning? And how is it related to Deep Learning or Neural Networks?

AI is developed with a goal to simulate human thinking and decision-making processes to perform complex tasks like object detection, speech recognition, natural language processing, to name a few. AI is the overall software system that automates the process, whereas machine learning is a subset of it which makes the decisions based on the data. Deep Learning is a specialized kind of machine learning, which makes inferences based on Neural Networks. Figure 2.8 provides a relationship between AI, ML, and DL.

AI is an integral part of our daily lives, powering various capabilities we often take for granted. Spelling and grammar correction in tools like Microsoft Word or Google Docs uses natural language processing to suggest improvements. Face recognition

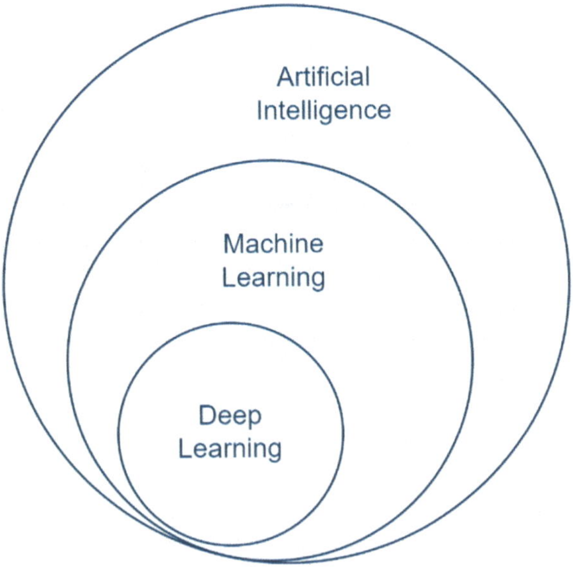

Fig. 2.8 Machine Learning and Deep Learning is a subset of AI

technology unlocks our phones using computer vision, while smart speakers like Alexa and Google Home rely on speech recognition to execute voice commands. Online shopping platforms use recommender systems to suggest personalized products based on browsing and purchase history. Additionally, banks leverage AI to detect fraudulent transactions by identifying anomalies in user behaviour. These examples highlight how advancements in AI, machine learning, and predictive capabilities, including Generative AI, are seamlessly embedded in the systems we use at home and work.

Generative AI (Gen AI)

Generative AI, as the name suggests, generates texts, images, and videos based on natural language inputs i.e. text, speech. The most popular application created with Generative AI is ChatGPT, which made AI so popular with common people from all fields, not only just people working in the tech industry. We are increasingly seeing so many applications of this, in the form of chatbots and so many other tools embedded in various applications we use developed on the foundations of the generative AI capabilities.

Generative AI uses Deep Learning capabilities and can be visualized as a subset of Deep Learning, as depicted in Fig. 2.9.

In Gen AI with simple instructions, called *prompts*, it is possible to generate what we need in the form of text, images, and videos. Here is a simple experiment, asking ChatGPT to generate names of ten largest countries with their capitals in a tabular format. We type in the text instructing ChatGPT to provide what we need,

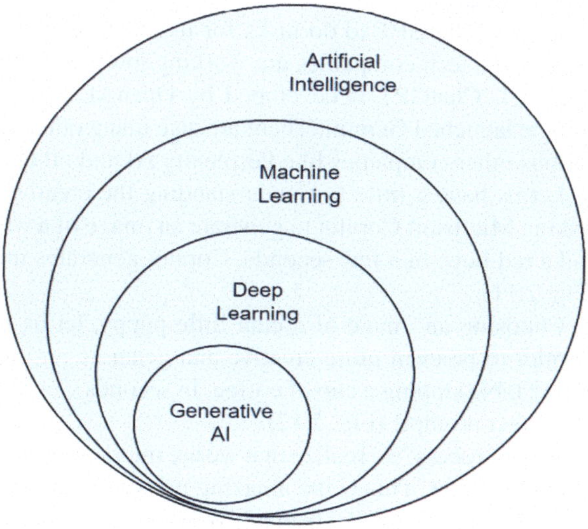

Fig. 2.9 Generative AI uses Deep Learning capabilities

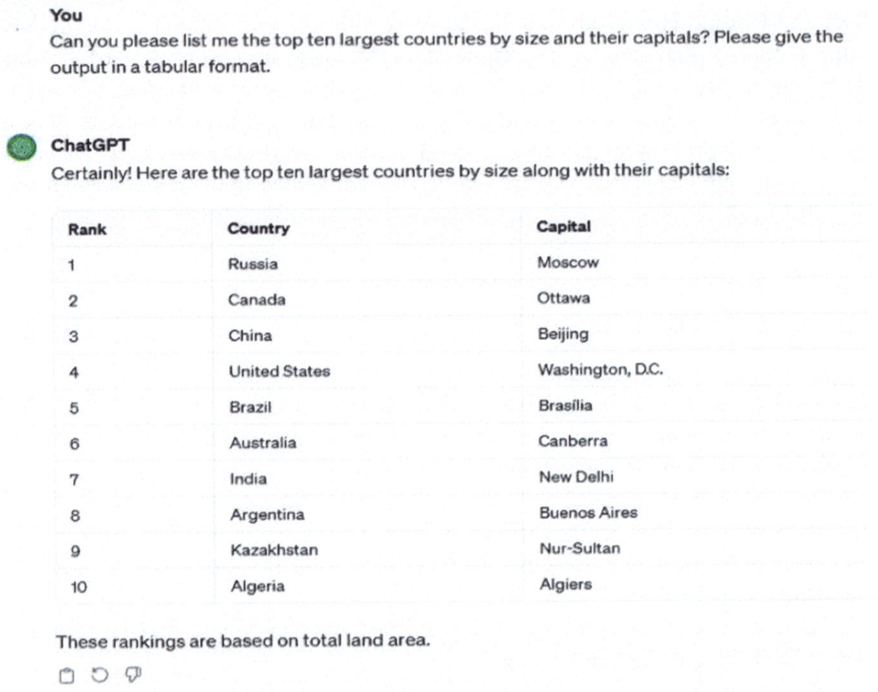

You

Can you please list me the top ten largest countries by size and their capitals? Please give the output in a tabular format.

ChatGPT

Certainly! Here are the top ten largest countries by size along with their capitals:

Rank	Country	Capital
1	Russia	Moscow
2	Canada	Ottawa
3	China	Beijing
4	United States	Washington, D.C.
5	Brazil	Brasília
6	Australia	Canberra
7	India	New Delhi
8	Argentina	Buenos Aires
9	Kazakhstan	Nur-Sultan
10	Algeria	Algiers

These rankings are based on total land area.

Fig. 2.10 ChatGPT generated table

and magically ChatGPT provides the output in seconds, formatted in the form of a table (Fig. 2.10).

Asking ChatGPT to do tasks for us increases our efficiency, and creativity too. Many large tech companies are working towards building these AI capabilities like ChatGPT. ChatGPT is developed by OpenAI, Microsoft has created Copilot and Google launched Gemini. There are also many other such capabilities being built by various other companies like Perplexity AI and others.

Let us have a little fun understanding the creative capability of Generative AI. Asking Microsoft Copilot to generate an image of a white puppy wearing sunglasses and a red bow. In a few seconds, Copilot generates images based on the text inputs (Fig. 2.11).

Choosing an image of a cute little puppy, let us have a little more fun, asking Copilot to be even more creative and generate an image of this puppy sitting at a dining table sipping a cup of coffee. In seconds Copilot provides an image requested in the text prompt! (Fig. 2.12).

In the process, we realize that we are interacting with the Copilot asking it to work as our assistant. This is the amazing power of Generative AI. But how does all this work? Under the hood of Generative AI are *Large Language Model*, also called *LLM*. Over the years a lot of development has happened in machine learning, and usage

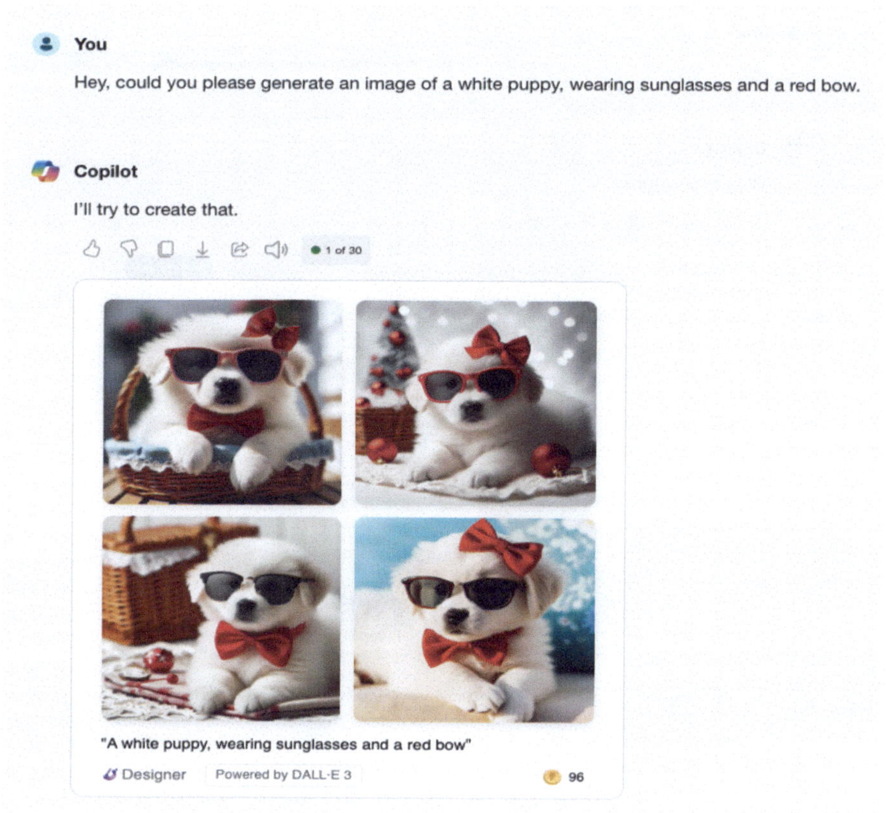

Fig. 2.11 Copilot generated images

of statistics and mathematical functions along with Natural language Processing to develop these Large Language Models.

Large Language Models (LLMs) are advanced machine learning models trained on massive datasets (corpora) to perform Natural Language Processing (NLP) tasks. These foundation models, such as GPT-4, Gemini, and LLaMA, can generate text, answer questions, translate languages, and summarize content. The input to these models is called a prompt, and crafting effective prompts is known as prompt engineering. Specialized LLMs, like Mental Lama for mental health, are trained on domain-specific datasets to perform targeted tasks.

LLMs work by predicting the next word in a sentence based on prior context. While they provide powerful results, they have limitations, such as outdated information and hallucinations—where outputs can be incorrect or unreal. Techniques like Retrieval Augmented Generation (RAG) connect LLMs to external data sources, enhancing accuracy. Despite their potential, LLMs require careful use, with risks and challenges addressed in ethical considerations.

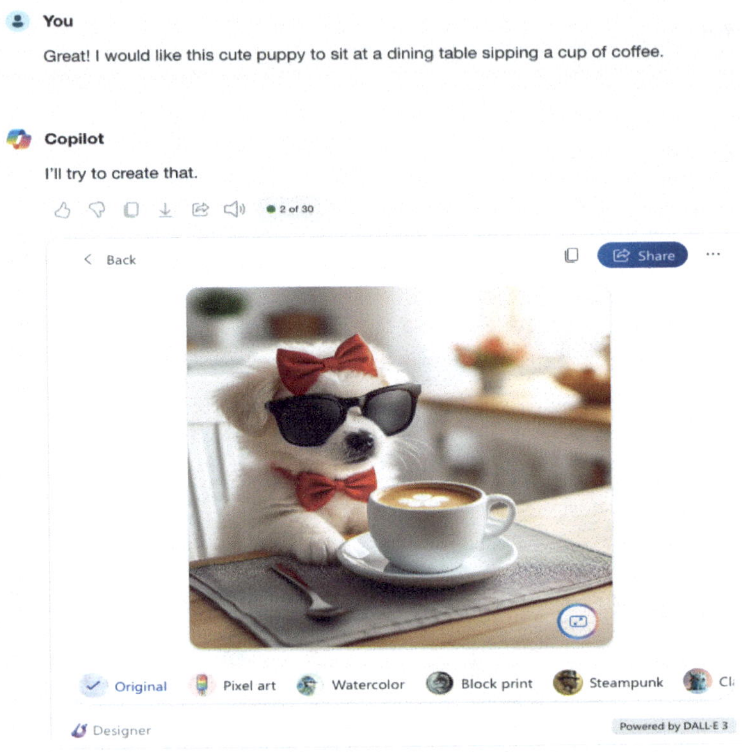

Fig. 2.12 Copilot generated images

Big Data

The success of AI applications is dependent on one critical component, *data*. Relevant and excellent quality data is the key ingredient for building successful machine learning models and AI applications. Real-world data is not always the perfect data to run machine learning algorithms. The data is often messy, has a lot of inconsistencies, and needs to be prepared before it may be used to train machine learning models. While *quality* of data is important, a vast *quantity* of data is also a necessity to train machine learning models. Real-world data are available in various forms, like audio, video, images, text and can be obtained from disparate sources, including organization databases, spreadsheets, social media, and public datasets made available by governments and institutions. For certain use cases data needs to be collected from various sources using forms, surveys, and even manually collecting the inputs (Fig. 2.13).

Let us look at an example scenario of an interaction between a doctor and patient to realize the amount of valuable data that gets generated. A patient uses an app or calls up the clinic to book an appointment with the doctor. The appointment is

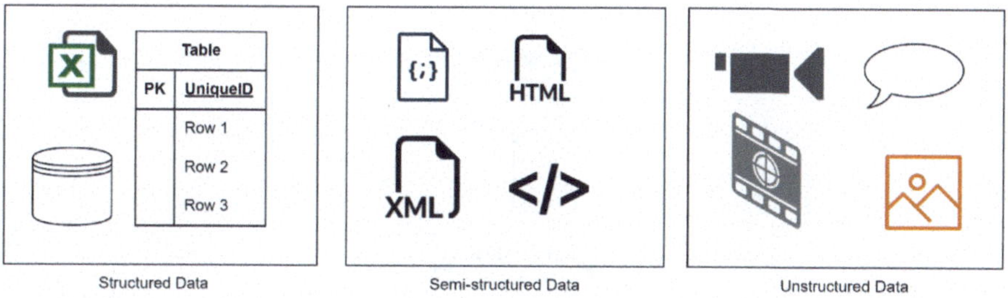

Fig. 2.13 Types of data

recorded in a database or spreadsheet, having various attributes like patient name, age, phone number, doctor's name, day, and time of appointment, repeat visit or first time visit, etc. During the appointment, the doctor does the investigation and records the observations, diagnosis, and writes a prescription. In recent times, clinics and hospitals often scan the prescription for medical records or the doctor often use the computer to record the details, like symptoms, observations, and prescribed medicines, and provide a print copy of the prescription to the patient. The prescriptions are available online and can be accessed with the right authorizations. This generates a vast amount of data in text or image form depending on the process followed. Let us assume that the doctor recommends some pathological tests and X-Ray. As the tests are performed, pathological tests' parametric data and X-ray images need to be stored in various systems. Apart from this there are financial transactions that are performed through card or cash and are recorded in various financial systems. This single instance of interaction generates this vast amount of data. Imagine this happening in many thousands of transactions daily.

Big data has these key characteristics (DT Editorial Services, n.d.):

1. Volume: It is the amount of data generated by individuals and organizations. The vast quantity of data is being generated every moment and it is growing exponentially. Data is being generated from all sources like social media, data within organizations, sensor data from millions of devices, emails, documents, YouTube videos, music files, and so on. This implies that there should be enough *storage* to store this large magnitude of data and capabilities to manage this large volume of data.
2. Velocity: The speed at which the data is being generated. The generated data needs to be processed in real-time and acted upon. For example, at the expressway toll gates the camera scans the toll tag on the car, deducts the toll charges from the consumers' account, and then the instruction is sent back to the toll gate assembly to open the barrier. This is happening every minute with tens of thousands of toll gates across the country with billions of ongoing transactions into various systems. Technology needs to be able to *ingest* such a large amount of data every second and there needs to be enough *compute power* to process this data in real-time. Another example is Google Maps, which has millions of datapoints generated from mobile devices every second and provides the drivers

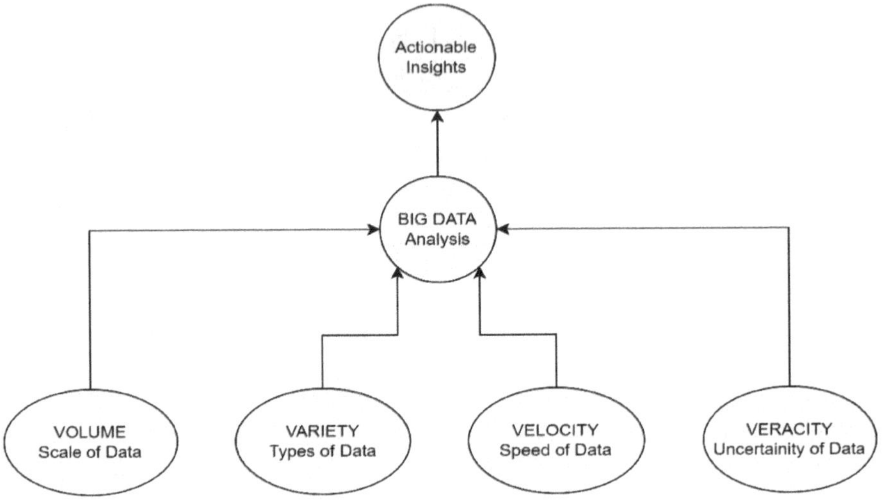

Fig. 2.14 Four Vs of Big Data

real-time updates on traffic and road conditions and calculating the fastest routes. To process this in near-real time not only do we need huge storage but massive computing power too.

3. Variety: Diverse types of data that are being generated every second. Diverse sources are generating several types of data starting from sensor data, video surveillance, photos, documents, audio, and so on. This warrants various technological capabilities to ingest, process, and store the data for further consumption.
4. Veracity: It is the uncertainty in the data, whether the data is consistent and correct. Pre-processing of the data is required to make it suitable for analysis. Correct data is key to gain actionable insights (Fig. 2.14).

Analysing and drawing inferences from this *big data* can lead to forecasting ability, actionable insights, and better decision-making. However, there are significant challenges in terms of storage, processing, and analysis due to its size and complexity. These data are often not in the format that is ready for analysis. Significant efforts are required to pre-process the data before it can be passed to machine learning models for learning and predicting. As a general estimate, for machine learning projects eighty per cent of the effort goes to acquiring and pre-processing the data and twenty per cent of the effort goes to development of the models. While improving the performance of the models, improving the quality and quantity of the data has a considerable influence, compared to the improvement that is achieved through fine-tuning the model parameters. There is a common terminology, *garbage in, garbage out*. This is so true for data-driven solutions.

Machine learning models tend to work well when there is a vast amount of data on which the model can be trained on. Also, the models need to be asked to draw inference from the same type of data. For example, let us assume that a model has been trained on particularly superior quality of X-Ray images to detect presence of COVID-19 in patients. Now, if the model is supplied with inferior quality X-Ray images for drawing inferences, it may not be able to detect COVID-19 correctly in the unseen samples. Also, machine learning models do not perform well when they are trained on lesser amounts of data. Often people believe that there is some data they have in spreadsheets and AI can do magic with that data, however that is not feasible. *Quality* and *quantity* of data is the key consideration when deciding on an AI use case. AI is not the magic wand for solving every problem. Careful considerations need to be made to decide if AI can be useful in each scenario.

Also, for machine learning solutions, machine learning models are not the only factor that needs to be considered. For training models lots of *Compute* resources are required along with large amount of *Storage* for storing the data. Considerable investments may be required, and estimations need to be made to check the financial viability of pursuing an AI project. There are techniques for cost optimization which need to be considered, discussion of which is beyond the scope of this book.

Dealing with data security, compliance and regulations are also of paramount importance. The data obtained often contain sensitive Personal Identifiable Information (PII), which can identify an individual like passports, driving licence, social security numbers, medical records, etc. Understanding PII is extremely important, and companies need to adhere to the laws and regulations required to protect individual's information. There are regulations like General Data Protection Regulation (GDPR) in EU, Health Insurance Portability and Accountability Act (HIPAA) in the healthcare industry, Sarbanes–Oxley Act (SOX) for financial data, Payment Card Industry Data Security Standard (PCI DSS) for credit card handling, and many more. These regulations guide data collection, storage, access, and sharing while ensuring compliance with existing laws and ethical standards. It is crucial for organizations and professionals to understand and adhere to these regulations when handling data. Failure to comply with these regulations can lead to severe penalties, both financially and reputationally. Data breaches are paramount, and careful considerations need to be made for securing the data and protecting individuals' safety and rights.

All these challenges need to be dealt with for building data-driven AI applications. Stakeholder investments, optimizing the costs, and managing the budget become a major factor that drives adoptability and sustainability of AI-based systems.

Big data analytics has transformed businesses and technology by enabling insights from large datasets to improve decision-making, predict trends, and optimize processes. It uncovers hidden patterns, relationships, and trends, driving strategies for better customer service, cost reduction, and competitive advantage. Modern technologies allow near-real-time analysis, providing instant insights, such as detecting fraudulent banking transactions. In health care, including mental health, big data analytics helps practitioners and patients by improving services and outcomes. Success in this field requires collaboration between healthcare professionals, IT experts, data scientists, and researchers to develop effective, domain-specific solutions for real-world applications (Fig. 2.15).

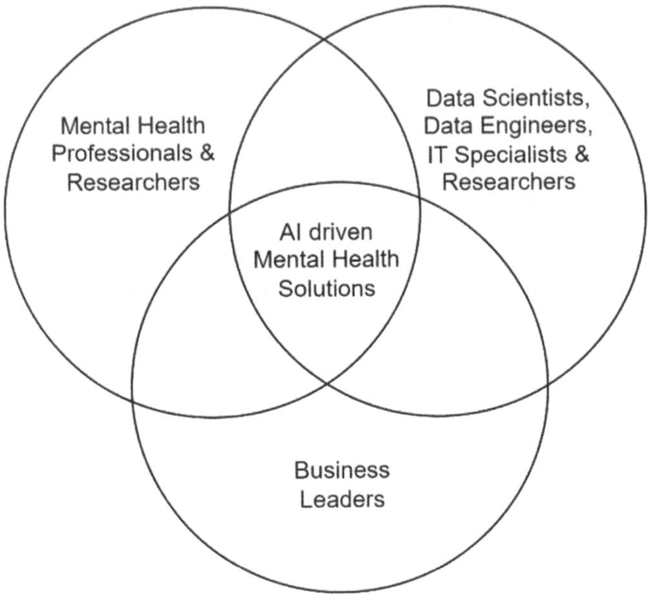

Fig. 2.15 Stakeholders of AI programmes

Big data analytics can be broadly classified into three types (DT Editorial Services, n.d.) of analytics:

1. Descriptive Analytics: This is based on the analysis of various features of the data and their correlations. In Data Science terminology, this is often called Exploratory Data Analysis. Descriptive analytics is important to understand the data, present historical findings. Based on these findings, decisions can be taken by the stakeholders.
2. Predictive Analytics: This is to forecast and predict based on the dataset. Statistical techniques, probability theory, and machine learning models are used for prediction.
3. Prescriptive Analytics: This prescribes what needs to be done based. This is based on the foundations of descriptive and predictive analytics, and various algorithms are used for prescriptive analytics based on the use cases.

Big Data Systems

Big data cannot be managed by traditional databases and systems. Specialized platforms have been developed to handle these massive amounts of data from disparate sources, which provide scalability and compute power to host analytical applications. These systems can ingest massive amounts of data at a very high-speed, store, pre-process, analyse, draw inferences, and present customized desired information and actionable insights to users and other downstream applications, in near real-time. This led to the development of technologies like Hadoop, Spark, High Performance Computing (HPC), Data warehouses, Data Lakes, and NoSQL databases. Architectures like Kappa and Lambda were developed to handle this kind of data. While the scope of this book would not make it possible to dive deeper into these technologies, the *Further Reading* section of the book lists resources on these topics for the interested reader.

In real-world use cases, there are two types of data processing that are required, *batch data processing* and *streaming data processing*.

Let us understand these terms by examples. There are twenty transactions that you did at your bank in a month, withdrawing money from the ATM, paying bills through the online application, depositing cheques, used the debit card at retail outlets, and transferred money to another bank account. All these transactions are stored in the banking system. At the month end, the bank processes all the transactional data in the system, consolidates it, and sends you a monthly statement. Here the transactions stored over the month are the batch data and batch data processing are performed to generate the monthly statements. However, banks also have systems running at the back-end, analysing every transaction to check if they are fraudulent transactions and perform the analysis in near real-time. This is stream data processing.

Batch data processing is defined as:

- Processing large amounts of data where a group of transactions is collected over a certain period.
- Data is collected, stored, pre-processed, and then analysed and output produced.
- Generally, data is sorted and processed in a sequential manner.
- There are fixed times when these batch jobs are scheduled and executed.
- Payroll, daily or weekly sales reports, monthly analysis of customer surveys are some examples of batch data processing systems.

Streaming data processing is defined as:

- Input, processing, and output of data happen on a continual basis.
- The analysis is typically completed in a few seconds, and output is produced for immediate consumption.
- Data is processed whenever there is input data ingested into the systems.
- IoT applications, real-time recommendation systems, online gaming, financial analysis are some of the examples of streaming data processing systems.

Let us look at a high-level schematic of how these systems work (Fig. 2.16).

1. Data Sources: These are the sources like sensors, mobile apps, tweets, social media posts, click stream data, online transactions, etc. that generate millions of data each second. These data sources communicate through some communication protocols with the back-end application hosted in the Cloud or in Data Centres. The number of data sources and the rate at which data is generated and needs to be received by the back-end system drive decisions on designing the architecture.

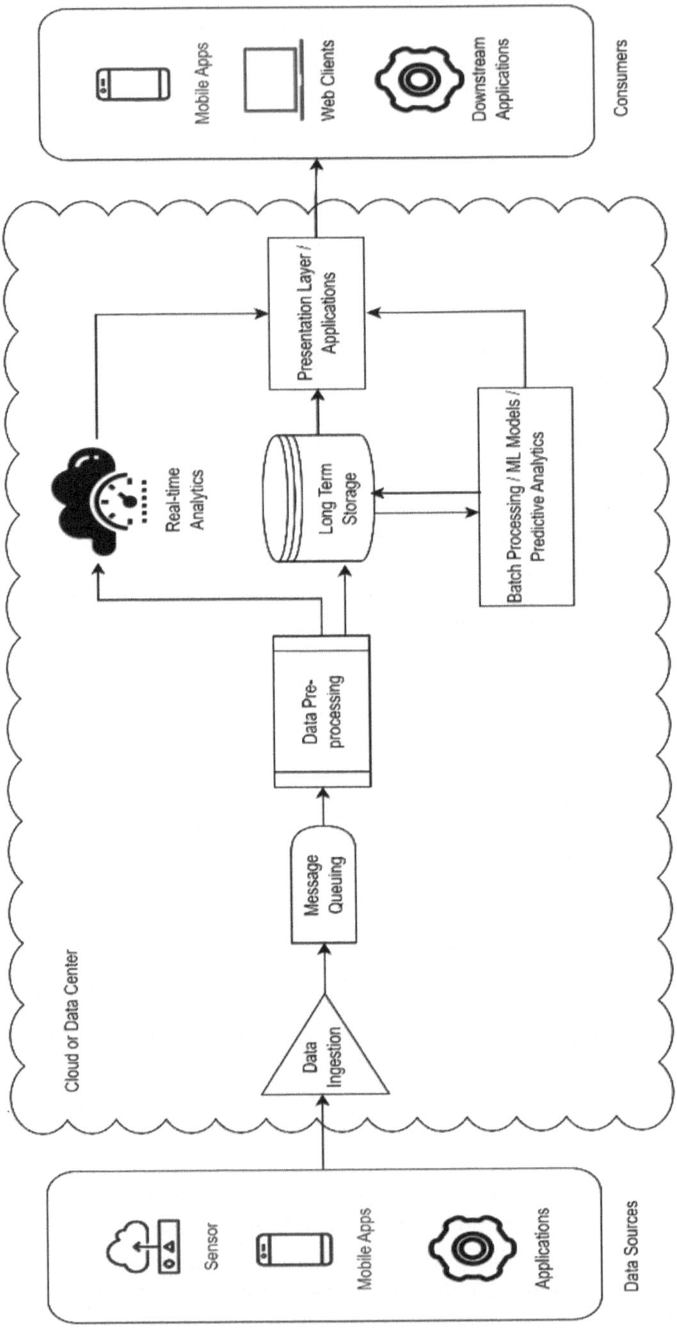

Fig. 2.16 Architecture of Streaming Systems

2. Data Ingestion: The data ingestion layer collects the data from the sources and ingests the data into the system for storage and analysis. Depending on the volume of data that is received the system should have redundancy built-in to be always available to accept the data. The system should have the scalability to ingest data based on the rate at which data sources generate the data.
3. Message Queueing: The rate at which data is ingested may be much faster than the speed at which it can be written to a storage system, like a database, or can be analysed in real-time by compute resources. The message queuing layer works as a buffer to allow the data to be stored and analysed without losing the data. There are technologies that do online processing and analysis of the incoming stream of data without permanently storing the data. These are design decisions that are considered based on the requirements.
4. Data Pre-processing: Real-world data is messy and may need to be cleaned and formatted to feed into machine learning models. The data pre-processing layer cleans and formats the data before sending for real-time analysis or long-term storage.
5. Real-time Analytics: Use cases and applications that need immediate analysis and output, like fraud detection systems for credit card transactions, analyse the streaming data in near real-time and send the output to a presentation layer or application. Under the hood of the real-time analytics systems are machine learning models that do the inferencing and generate an output.
6. Long-term Storage: The data in raw and processed forms, as well as the outputs are stored in long-term storages, like databases and data lakes. This is used for batch processing and further analytics and is sent to the presentation layer for consumption.
7. Batch Processing/ML Models/Predictive Analytics: This is the layer where batch processing is performed on the data and machine learning models do the inference and produce the required output.
8. Presentation Layer/Applications: This layer hosts the applications that are consumed by the consumers. The outputs could be presented through custom applications, APIs, or output files. The interface accessed through browsers or mobile apps is hosted in this layer.
9. Consumers: Depending on the use cases the output is consumed by users or other applications. These may be consumer applications or other applications that take this as an input for further processing and presentation.

As we have observed, there are many moving parts that come together to build an analytics system. For a well-architected analytics system, the following are the key considerations (Amazon Web Services, 2023) for building and running reliable, secure, efficient, cost-effective, and sustainable systems:

1. Operational Excellence: Support the systems efficiently for development and maintenance, with full observability of the environment and continual improvement of processes and procedures to run the systems.
2. Security: Protect the systems and sensitive data from bad actors and prevent data leakages.

3. Reliability: The systems should continue to be available and serve the intended purpose consistently.
4. Performance Efficiency: Maintain the performance of the systems and deliver the outcomes within the intended response times.
5. Cost Optimization: Keep the costs down as much as possible without compromising on the other parameters.
6. Sustainability: Goal to reduce the energy consumption of the resources and minimize the carbon footprint.

Cloud

The architecture discussed above needs to be hosted somewhere. There are broadly two options, either in a data centre on-premises (provided by a colocation provider or owned by the organization developing the systems) or use the Cloud services from one of the Cloud Service Providers.

Challenges of hosting the infrastructure in the datacentres are many, and often hosting the solutions with the Cloud Service Providers may be more suitable for many organizations. Before we go deeper into discussing the pros and cons of hosting at the data centre or in the Cloud, let us review what Cloud is.

In 2011, National Institute of Standards and Technology (NIST), US Department of Commerce, published *The NIST Definition of Cloud Computing* (Mell & Grance, 2011). The report defines the five essential characteristics of Cloud:

1. On-demand Self-service: Consumers can create the required services on their own without the need of any human support from the service providers. Consumers use the Cloud Services portal to create their own login, include the billing information with their own credit card details and create the resources and services.
2. Broad Network Access: The service should be available from anywhere using the internet and should be accessible using any platforms, e.g. laptops, mobile phones, tablets, etc.
3. Resource Pooling: The consumer uses the compute, storage, network, and other resources from an available pool of resources, which are shared by multiple customers. Once a resource is no longer required and released by a customer, it is released back to the pool and is available for the other customers.
4. Rapid Elasticity: Based on demand, the resources and services can be scaled up or down, with automation capabilities. The cloud services have enough resources available in the pool for large scale deployments, and rarely availability of resources is a constraint.
5. Measured Service: Resource usage is monitored, controlled, and reported and consumers are billed transparently based on consumption.

The report discusses the three Service Models of the Cloud:

- Software as a Service (SaaS)
- Platform as a Service (PaaS)

– Infrastructure as a Service (IaaS).

It also defines four Deployment Models for the Cloud:

– Private Cloud
– Community Cloud
– Public Cloud
– Community Cloud.

For the interested reader, the details are available in the paper and not covered in the scope of this book. The Cloud that is used by most consumers is the Public Cloud. The three prominent Cloud Service Providers are:

– Amazon Web Services (AWS)—https://aws.amazon.com
– Microsoft Azure (Azure)—https://azure.microsoft.com
– Google Cloud Platform (GCP)—https://cloud.google.com

All these Cloud Service Providers provide technologies and services to build scalable and reliable platforms to host data intensive, machine learning, and analytics applications.

While we discussed Cloud and the Public Cloud Service providers, the analytics applications can also be hosted on-premises, in the organization's own data centre or at a colocation space providing facilities to keep the equipment. Many large organizations own data centres and can host the workloads on-premises, however there are some challenges that one should be aware of.

Here are some of the challenges of hosting on-premises:

1. Capital Expenditure: Significant investment is required to build the infrastructure and would need to be paid upfront or leased. In the Cloud, the starting cost could be low, and one pays for what one uses without any upfront capital expenditure.
2. Capacity Planning and Idle Resources: In on-premises it will be required to plan for the peak-capacity to ensure there is no impact to the services, however if these resources may not always be required and be idle. Cloud allows for inward and outward scalability, and one pays for the consumed resources only.
3. Operational Costs: Maintenance of on-premises environments may need additional expenditures like rents, electricity charges, staff salaries for managing the datacentre and equipment, security, insurance, and taxes. Cloud would need skilled staff to focus on the application development and maintenance, eliminating the overheads needed to maintain an on-premises environment.
4. Reliability, Uptime, and Disaster Recovery: Significant planning, effort, and costs are required to maintain the infrastructure for reliability and additional locations for disaster recovery.

Careful consideration should be made between the choice of hosting applications on-premises or in the Cloud depending on several factors, and most importantly on the current state. A holistic review is required with Total Cost of Ownership (TCO) analysis to determine which is the most suitable approach to consider.

Applications of AI

AI can be used in various use cases. Broadly these are the applications of AI which are applied in various real-world use cases.

Natural Language Processing: Natural Language Processing (NLP) is a segment within AI that interprets text and speech. There are many applications of AI which are used heavily in many applications today. Some of the use cases are:

- Language Translation to translate from one language to another
- Sentiment analysis identifies the sentiment of the text. Often used to track social media posts and reviews to understand the sentiment about the comments consumers make about a product.
- Summarization is often used for summarizing documents
- Named identity recognition identifies places, people, organizations, etc. Within the corpus of text
- Detect Personally Identifiable Information (PII) within a corpus.
- Key phrase extraction extracts key points from within a text document.
- Speech-to-Text and Text-to-Speech conversions.

Computer Vision: Computer vision uses Deep Learning and Convolution Neural Network (CNN) to perform various tasks. Some of the common uses of Computer Vision are:

- In the healthcare domain for detecting diseases from X-Rays, MRIs, and other images
- Facial detection in smartphones and photo apps
- Surveillance systems to detect any intruders in video frames
- Self-driving cars use it for detecting traffic signals, other cars, and pedestrians
- In the agriculture domain to detect the health of crops.

These are some examples of what can be achieved through AI. These technologies can be adopted in various situations to automate various tasks.

AI and Retail: AI has become a powerful tool in logistics, supply chain, and transportation, rapidly transforming these industries. With vast amounts of data accumulated over years, the use of AI and machine learning now enables advanced analysis, optimization, and real-time decision-making. Predictive analytics can foresee transportation needs, helping avoid delays and breakdowns. Strategic optimization allows for faster, data-driven decisions. Robotics is utilized in warehouses for inventory tracking and movement, while autonomous vehicles are set to revolutionize logistics by reducing labour costs and improving efficiency.

AI and Agriculture: In agriculture, AI enhances productivity and efficiency, tackling issues such as climate change and food security. Precision agriculture leverages technologies like GPS, drones, and sensors to enable accurate monitoring and management of crops. AI applications include agricultural robots for planting and harvesting, crop and soil monitoring systems like the Plantix app for soil health assessment, and predictive analytics to forecast weather impacts on crop yield. This integration of AI helps farmers optimize resource use and boost crop productivity.

AI and Health Care: AI's impact on health care is substantial, aiding in diagnosis, treatment, and patient care. Decision support systems analyse large datasets to assist doctors in making faster, more accurate decisions. AI tools can highlight abnormalities in patient scans, improving diagnosis accuracy. Chatbots and apps collect patient data, alleviating physician workload and reducing burnout. In diagnostics, deep learning algorithms help detect conditions like cancer, while facial recognition software identifies genetic disorders. Additionally, AI supports robotic surgeries, enhancing precision and reducing recovery time. The use of AI in drug discovery is accelerating, as machine learning identifies potential drug candidates efficiently, reducing the time and cost of development.

Risks and Challenges

While AI offers numerous benefits, it also poses significant risks and challenges. Data privacy and security are critical concerns, as vast amounts of sensitive data, including Personally Identifiable Information (PII), must be securely stored to prevent breaches, such as in healthcare or retail transactions. Bias in training data, such as demographic or gender bias, can lead to unfair and inaccurate model outcomes. Responsible AI is essential to mitigate risks of generating harmful or toxic content, particularly in Generative AI and Large Language Models, requiring thorough testing during development. Additionally, explainable AI is vital in sensitive domains like health care and finance, ensuring practitioners and consumers can understand and trust AI-driven decisions.

There is a separate Chapter on Managing Data Privacy and Security, Ethics and Considerations of AI exploring these risks and challenges in greater detail.

References

Amazon Web Services. (2023). *AWS well-architected framework whitepaper*. Amazon Web Services, Inc. https://docs.aws.amazon.com/pdfs/wellarchitected/latest/framework/wellarchitected-framework.pdf

DT Editorial Services. (n.d.). Getting an overview of big data. In DT Editorial Services (Ed.), *Big data black book (2019)*. Dreamtech Press.

Jaber, N. (2022, March 22). Can artificial intelligence help see cancer in new, and better, ways? *National Cancer Institute*. https://www.cancer.gov/news-events/cancer-currents-blog/2022/artificial-intelligence-cancer-imaging

Maslej, N., Fattorini, L., Brynjolfsson, E., Etchemendy, J., Ligett, K., Lyons, T., Manyika, J., Ngo, H., Niebles, J. C., Parli, V., Shoham, Y., Wald, R., Clark, J., & Perrault, R. (2023). *The AI Index 2023 Annual Report*. AI Index Steering Committee, Institute for Human-Centered AI, Stanford University. https://aiindex.stanford.edu

Mell, P. M., & Grance, T. (2011). *The NIST Definition of Cloud Computing*. https://doi.org/10.6028/NIST.SP.800-145

Chapter 3
Bringing AI and Mental Health Together

Abstract Awareness regarding mental health has gained prominence in recent years, and there has been a welcome increase in stakeholders' efforts to enhance the efficacy of existing treatment approaches, make them more customized to patients, while addressing socio-cultural factors. As Artificial Intelligence (AI) makes inroads in almost all services including health, mental health cannot be left behind. Compared to other medical fields, there is relatively lesser presence of lab-based tests in diagnostic and management of mental health issues. Thus, it is intriguing to understand if AI has reliable implications in mental health services, and if implemented can bring significant change in enhancing efficiency of services and empowering professionals. The present chapter provides a backdrop of AI essentials and their possible utilization in mental health.

Keyword Natural language processing · Decision-making · Early identification · Mental health care

Overview

The conventional approach to manage mental health issues include the pharmacological and non-pharmacological interventions. Both are anchored on a clinical diagnosis made by trained professionals and rely heavily on clinical history. Irrespective of the approach, an effective communication between client and the therapist is important, and unlike other medical fields, there are no lab-based diagnostic tests for mental ill health conditions. In such a scenario, it is obvious to have apprehensions whether and how much AI can be integrated in these processes in mental health services. However, the convergence of AI and mental health is becoming increasingly prominent, offering innovative solutions to address significant challenges in the process.

AI primarily focuses on developing systems with human-like intelligence, enabling them to handle tasks like problem-solving and decision-making. As we speak of merging AI and mental health, the application of AI techniques, including

S. Halder et al., *Navigating AI in Mental Health Care*,
https://doi.org/10.1007/978-981-96-9744-1_3

machine learning, natural language processing, and data analytics, become prominent in advancing mental health care. These technologies have the potential to revolutionize how we diagnose, treat, and provide support for mental health issues, improving efficiency, scalability, and accessibility. At the same time, this intersection also raises important concerns regarding ethics and privacy, such as data security, algorithmic bias, and depersonalization. Recognizing the synergy between AI and mental health is essential as it holds the promise of enhancing mental healthcare and potentially reducing the burden of mental health disorders on individuals and society. To ensure that AI positively impacts mental health, it is crucial to implement it responsibly while taking ethical considerations into account. This chapter delves into the implications and significance of this intersection. For laymen, it might be difficult to comprehend how AI can be used to engage in tasks conventionally done by trained clinicians. Let's explore fundamental AI techniques and their applications in advancing mental health care:

Machine Learning (ML): It is a type of AI that enables algorithms to autonomously learn from data to perform well-defined tasks and make future predictions. Layman people may wonder how a software programme can predict about a person's chances to develop a certain illness. Well, the idea is to see patterns in the data of an individual, which could be genetic history, certain scans of the human brain, specific birth, and developmental history or other measurable data that are risk factors for the development of a mental ill health condition. So, higher number of risk factors would indicate higher probability of developing the specific disorder. This may sound like science fantasy, and there also might be some scope of error, but machine learning is meant to improve as more and more data is chipped in.

Either way in mental health precautions is always better, and primary prevention is always considered to be the best strategy. Thus, machine learning algorithms can analyse patient data to predict mental health risks for diagnosis and Risk Prediction. One of the major works prominently cited for use of AI is in early detection of risk is in the domain of suicide risk and depression, where researchers have used machine learning to predict the likelihood of depression based on social media posts or user behaviour patterns (Ryu et al., 2019; Linthicum et al., 2019; Castillo et al. 2020). An advantage of unbiased analysis of patient data through machine learning is that it can analyse patient responses to different therapies and medications, aiding in personalized treatment recommendations. An example is using machine learning to predict which type of therapy might be most effective for an individual based on their characteristics and history. However, these advancements are in the preliminary stage, yet with too much potential (Chen et al. 2020; Lewanowicz et al., 2022).

Natural Language Processing (NLP): Natural language processing and sentiment analysis are extensively used to analyse text data from various sources, like social media, therapy transcripts, etc. to gauge emotional states of clients or healthy individuals. For instance, sentiment analysis can detect signs of distress or depressive tendencies in written communication. NLP techniques are instrumental and power conversational agents or chatbots that provide immediate support. These tools use language understanding to interact with users, offering guidance or assistance. For example, Woebot is an AI chatbot designed to provide cognitive-behavioural therapy techniques to its users.

Data Analytics: Data analytics is an important tool primarily meant for analysing raw data and explaining why the data followed a particular pattern; what could be the likely course taken by the data, and what actions should be taken. In nutshell it recognizes patterns and data analytics in mental health involves spotting patterns in large datasets. For example, analysing electronic health records of patients can reveal correlations between certain behaviours or environmental factors and mental health outcome intervention by analysing behavioural data. Data analytics can help in early identification of potential mental health issues. For example, analysis of smartphone usage patterns might help detect early signs of conditions like bipolar disorder or schizophrenia, in individuals at risk. Thus, AI techniques are proving handy not only for diagnosis and treatment but also for prevention and ongoing support in mental health care. However, it's essential to ensure data privacy, accuracy, and ethical considerations in deploying these AI-driven solutions in such sensitive areas.

Artificial intelligence, as a constantly evolving field, focuses on developing systems with human-like intelligence, enabling them to handle tasks like problem-solving and decision-making. It strives to create systems that can mimic human intelligence to some degree. As mentioned earlier, problem-solving, decision-making, learning, and understanding natural language are some key areas, which AI endeavours to replicate or augment with machine capabilities. As the field progresses, the researchers' aim is to make AI systems more adaptable, efficient, and capable of handling complex tasks across various domains. This pursuit involves several key aspects:

Replicating Human-like Intelligence: AI aims to simulate human cognitive abilities such as reasoning, learning, perception, problem-solving, and decision-making. Through algorithms, models, and data processing, AI systems attempt to mimic the way humans analyse information and make choices. It is very human to be apprehensive to lose control over and be overpowered by something created by us only. However, it's not going to happen, as the basic idea of using AI in mental health care is to help professionals in better decision-making rather than letting AI make decisions.

Problem-solving Capabilities: AI systems are designed to tackle complex problems across various domains. They utilize algorithms, heuristics, and learning mechanisms to explore solutions and optimize outcomes. For instance, in health care, AI helps diagnose diseases by analysing symptoms and medical records, akin to how a human doctor would approach a diagnosis.

Decision-making Processes: AI systems endeavour to emulate human decision-making by processing vast amounts of data and using predefined rules or learned patterns to make informed choices. This can be seen in financial markets, where AI algorithms analyse market trends to suggest investment strategies. The same principles can be used in mental healthcare processes too with customization.

Learning and Adaptation: A significant facet of AI involves machine learning and its subsets like supervised, unsupervised, and reinforcement learning. These techniques enable systems to learn from data, refine their models, and adapt to new information or changing environments. This capability is crucial for AI systems to continuously improve their performance.

Natural Language Processing (NLP): Mentioned earlier too, NLP is a vital AI component that aims to comprehend and generate human language. Natural language processing techniques allow machines to understand, interpret, and respond to human language in a way that's meaningful and contextually relevant. NLP helps in understanding and analysing textual data, like therapy session transcripts or social media posts, to gauge mental states or emotional distress. Applications like chatbots, language translation, and sentiment analysis rely on NLP. However, NLP needs refinement to understand the actual essence of communication and may miss to understand sarcasm.

Ethical and Responsible AI Development

As AI progresses, there is a growing emphasis on developing ethical AI systems that align with societal values and principles. Ensuring fairness, transparency, and accountability in AI decision-making processes is crucial to foster trust and acceptance.

Continual Advancements: AI is a field marked by ongoing advancements. Innovations in neural networks, deep learning architectures, reinforcement learning, and other areas continue to enhance the capabilities of AI systems, making them more proficient at handling complex tasks. The journey towards creating AI systems with human-like intelligence involves a multidisciplinary approach encompassing computer science, mathematics, cognitive science, neuroscience, and ethics. While complete replication of human intelligence remains a distant goal, AI continues to progress, bringing significant advancements and transformative changes across various industries and domains.

We have already discussed mental health in the previous chapter and its significance in our lives. Mental health encompasses a broad spectrum of emotional and psychological well-being crucial for our overall wellness. It involves how we think, feel, and act, impacting our daily lives and interactions. Two very common prevalent conditions within this realm are depression and anxiety, but mental health is not limited to these alone. Depression is more than just feeling sad; it often involves persistent feelings of hopelessness, loss of interest in activities, changes in appetite or sleep, and difficulty concentrating. Anxiety, on the other hand, involves excessive worry, fear, or apprehension, which can manifest in physical symptoms like restlessness, irritability, muscle tension, and difficulty controlling worry.

These conditions, among others, significantly impact one's quality of life. Mental health concerns can stem from various factors, including genetic predispositions, life experiences, trauma, biological factors, or a combination of these elements. Recognizing the importance of mental health is crucial today. Destigmatizing these conditions and promoting open conversations encourage seeking help without judgement. Just as we care for our physical health, nurturing our mental well-being is essential for leading fulfilling lives. The significance of mental health has gained substantial attention for several reasons:

Increased Awareness and Advocacy: There's been a concerted effort to raise awareness about mental health, reducing stigma, and encouraging conversations around it. This has led to a better understanding of mental health issues and the importance of seeking help.

Stressful Modern Lifestyles: The pace of life has accelerated, leading to higher stress levels due to factors like work pressures, financial challenges, social expectations, and information overload. These stressors significantly impact mental well-being.

Pandemic Impact: The COVID-19 pandemic has intensified mental health concerns globally. Isolation, uncertainty, grief, economic instability, and disruptions to daily life have taken a toll on people's mental health, amplifying the need for support and resources.

Digital Influence: The prevalence of social media and digital technologies has altered social interactions and led to concerns about issues like cyberbullying, comparison-driven anxiety, and constant connectivity, affecting mental health negatively for some individuals.

Accessibility to Information: More accessible information has empowered individuals to recognize symptoms and seek help. Mental health education through various media has increased awareness about the importance of mental well-being.

Acknowledgements of Holistic Health: There's a growing recognition that overall health includes mental, emotional, and physical aspects. Holistic approaches to wellness have gained traction, emphasising the need to prioritize mental health for a balanced life.

Thus, there is no denial that mental health significantly affects productivity, relationships, and overall societal well-being. Recognizing and addressing mental health concerns can lead to more engaged, productive individuals and healthier communities. Given these factors, addressing mental health concerns has become a priority. Governments, organisations, and individuals are increasingly investing in mental health resources, support systems, and initiatives to ensure that mental well-being receives the attention and care it deserves.

Merging of AI and Mental Health

As we speak about the convergence of Artificial Intelligence and mental health, it appears as if the use of AI in the health sector is very novel. To the matter of fact, the early work on use of AI in the health sector dates back to the early 1960's. In 1972, researchers developed Internist-1, a system containing a knowledge base of causal and taxonomic relationships between clinical findings and diagnostic hypotheses, that used a powerful ranking algorithm to reach diagnoses. It represented a major shift in AI in clinical research because it had clear potential to take some of the onus of clinical diagnosis from healthcare providers and provided a mechanism for physicians to cross-check their differential diagnoses (Hirani et al., 2024). The use of AI in the health sector has grown and advanced multiple times since then; however, much of the available literature suggests its use mostly in the field of diagnostic imaging, genetics, electro diagnosis, screening, and evaluation. AI has generated immense potential for its use in detection, diagnosis, predicting progress in cardiac illness and cancer as well as improving accidents and emergency services. While the use of AI in different fields of health has evolved in a contemporary manner, much of the literature on use of AI specific to mental health started emerging in the mid-1980s only and have come into prominence only in the last ten years or so. One of the reasons behind this might be the lack of objective diagnostic measures in mental health compared to other fields of medicine, as there are no laboratory-based tests which can give diagnosis regarding mental ill health conditions. Further the non-pharmacological interventions and assessments in terms of psychological assessments, counselling and psychotherapy always had been one to one between the therapist and the client, even if using computerized or online formats. It would not be wrong to say that despite having diagnostic and treatment guidelines, there always has been an inherent hesitation both on part of clients and professionals to rely on machines and algorithms to understand the complex human mind and psyche.

Thus, when we speak of convergence of AI and mental health, it comes with a lot of apprehensions and doubts, whether this convergence is at all possible, and if yes, to what extent.

The use of any form of technology in health care, starting with the simplest to the most advanced ones primarily aim to enhance accuracy and assist in clinical diagnosis, ease professional human labour, to explore which could be difficult to discern for the human eyes and hands of the professional, to maintain critical data, to ease communication between client and therapist and provide access to clients in remote places to name a few.

Now, how do these objectives fit in the case of AI and Mental health? We must understand that treatment and management of mental ill health conditions are still an evolving domain with updates and changes in diagnostic classifications and categories still happening, which will continue in future too. The US classificatory systems for psychiatric disorders, the DSM has undergone several revisions since its introduction with all good intentions. However, it has also led to certain debate over the way the criterions for several disorders have been modified, especially in the latest version DSM 5. Many new diagnoses have been introduced, that are contended to be no more than severe variants of normal behaviour. On the other hand, certain existing conditions have been shifted or included into altogether new categories. It is remarkable to note that prevalence of certain diagnosed childhood psychiatric disorders has increased dramatically in recent decades. This increase is not mere 5 or 10 per cent, but significantly many fold. For example, the attention-deficit/hyperactivity disorder (ADHD) has tripled in rates in the past two–three decades; autistic disorders have increased by more than 20-fold. This hints towards the tendency or the pattern of overdiagnosis among professionals, caused by multiple factors, and some of them could be unintentional bias, error in clinical judgement, gap in communication between client and the mental health professional. This can be certainly improved, and AI can be effectively used in clinical decision-making that can help in better diagnostic processes.

Here we need to look into the conventional process of client consultation and management which happens in mental health and illness conditions. The process of diagnosing an individual with mental ill health condition, typically includes history taking, mental status examination or clinical interview in simple words and psychological assessment. The information gathered from all these is analysed by trained mental health professionals to filter relevant information to fit into one or more diagnostic criteria as per standard classificatory systems like the DSM or the ICD. The history taking and clinical interview may appear like a formal conversation between the client and the mental health professional; but in actual it is a professional task and carries maximum weightage in the diagnostic process. The process requires specific information on part of the client including but not limited to the primary concerns of the client, how the symptoms evolved and have progressed, the circumstances around the client before and during the evolution of the symptoms, personal and childhood history, and current mental status. It is very likely that clients focus more on their concerning problems and may skip something not important to them, but potentially important piece of information for the clinician. Reliability and adequacy of the information are always a concern during this process topped by potential subjective bias on part of the clinician. Thus, this is an important domain where AI can help clinicians in improving the diagnostic impressions.

On similar lines if we talk about the psychological interventions in mental health, namely psychotherapy and counselling, we see that there are numerous evidenced-based therapies for mental health conditions. However, unlike pharmacological interventions, psychotherapy is a time-taking procedure and involves frequent sessions with the therapist. Even though the therapy process is a professional work, there lie individual differences in therapists, in terms of their own orientation, competency over particular disorders, which may affect the therapeutic outcome. Language capabilities, psychological sophistication as well as cultural differences may also affect the therapeutic outcome. AI can be very handy in the therapeutic process as a facilitator and administrative assistant for record keeping, profiling, as well as tracking progress of the clients.

AI technologies are being utilized in various ways to enhance assessment, diagnosis, treatment, and support systems for individuals with mental health issues. Here are a few ways AI is making an impact in mental health care:

Early Detection and Diagnosis: As mentioned earlier primary prevention, or even secondary prevention are considered ideal when aiming for a favourable treatment outcome in mental health. In both these domains AI has huge implications, as AI algorithms can analyse patterns in behaviour, speech, or writing to identify early signs of mental health disorders. For instance, natural language processing (NLP) can analyse text or speech to detect changes that might indicate depression or anxiety. Further machine learning technologies can analyse vast amounts of data, including behavioural patterns, genetic information, and biometric data, to identify early signs of mental health issues. Predictive analytics can aid in recognizing potential risks and triggers. One of the major plus points of using AI in preventive measures for mental health would be, it could be free of any stigma that is associated, though not warranted, when an individual consults a mental health professional even for screening purposes. Even though lab-based tests, e.g. blood analysis or imaging, are not used currently for diagnosing mental ill health conditions; with large data made available there might be the possibility of building a unique profile of individuals who are at risk of developing mental ill health conditions. Wearable devices and smartphone applications can track subtle changes in behaviour, sleep patterns, heart rate, or speech patterns, providing objective data for early detection and diagnosis.

Improved Treatment Approaches: The treatment guidelines for most mental ill health conditions suggest a collaborative approach of psychiatrists, clinical psychologists, social workers, and other rehabilitation professionals as required. However, many times it is not possible because of unavailability of professionals under one roof or due to lack of coordination among different professionals. AI can be effectively used in the existing technologies to improve treatment approaches and outcomes. Like Telehealth and Teletherapy. Even though these technologies are not essentially AI; it can make the existing technologies more efficient. Virtual platforms enable people to access therapy and counselling remotely, breaking down geographical barriers and making mental health care more accessible. Similarly, Virtual Reality (VR) technology offers immersive environments for exposure therapy, helping individuals confront and manage phobias, post-traumatic stress, or anxiety disorders in a controlled and safe setting.

Mobile Apps and Online Program**me**s: These are primarily meant to provide insight about one's condition, self-help tools, and referral services for screening and consultation. The advanced-level apps also provide cognitive-behavioural therapy exercises, meditation guides, mood tracking, offering personalized support between therapy sessions. There is a wide range of Chatbots and Virtual Assistants that are specifically developed to cater mental health needs of users. AI-powered chatbots and virtual assistants offer immediate support by providing resources, guidance, and even therapeutic conversations. One of the good parts about chatbots is that these systems are available 24/7, providing accessibility and anonymity, which can encourage individuals to seek help any time. AI-driven applications provide accessible mental health support, breaking barriers of geographical distance and financial constraints. Chatbots and virtual assistants offer immediate help, guiding individuals through coping strategies or simply lending a listening ear. This constant availability can be crucial for individuals needing immediate support.

Supporting Professionals: AI can assist mental health professionals by sharing and automating administrative tasks, which allows them to focus more on direct patient care. It also aids in data analysis, helping professionals make more informed decisions about patient care. By analysing patterns and trends in data, algorithms can predict potential relapses or deteriorations in mental health, enabling proactive interventions on part of mental health professionals. While smart devices have been around for quite a time, they can be integrated with AI to be more effective and provide vital role in monitoring and support. Smart devices can offer real-time monitoring and alerts for caregivers or healthcare providers about changes in a person's behaviour or mental state. Wearable devices and smartphone applications integrated with AI can monitor behavioural patterns, sleep, activity levels, and even physiological signals. They can provide real-time feedback or alerts to individuals or their caregivers about changes that might indicate a decline in mental health. The smart devices have also enhanced remote access and connectivity of professionals with their clients. Technologies like the internet, mobile devices, and telecommunication tools have made information and services accessible from almost anywhere. This accessibility is particularly impactful in remote or underserved areas where traditional services might be limited. Efficient use of resources through technology is also cost effective and can significantly reduce costs. For instance, remote consultations in healthcare save travel expenses for patients and reduce infrastructure costs for healthcare providers.

Another benefit is in terms of scalability of services. When provided through cloud computing they allow for flexible and scalable solutions. Organizations can easily scale up or down their computing resources based on demand, enabling them to handle increased workloads without major infrastructure changes.

Personalized Treatment: Till date personalized treatment was mostly heard in terms of customized medication which were made on the basis of an individual's genetic and other biological profile. Therapeutic management in mental health is either way personalized as the therapeutic need of every client is different owing to their unique psychosocial background. However, these customizations may miss a few clues, which can be gained from data analysis. AI can assist in creating personalized treatment plans by analysing vast amounts of data from patients, considering individual differences and responses to specific therapies. This personalization can lead to more effective and tailored treatment options. AI can be utilized to process vast amounts of data from different sources, e.g. genetic, environmental, or behavioural to create personalized treatment plans. Genetic testing in particular and analysis can help personalize treatment plans, allowing for more targeted medication and therapies based on an individual's genetic makeup. Further machine learning models can be implemented to predict the effectiveness of different therapies for specific individuals, enabling tailored interventions.

Data Analysis for Insight and Research:

Technology facilitates global collaboration, allowing experts from different parts of the world to work together, share knowledge, and innovate collectively, thus fostering progress and development on a global scale. AI helps researchers analyse large datasets from various sources to identify broader trends in mental health and to discover new insights into mental health disorders, treatment effectiveness, and predictive models. This aids in developing better interventions and understanding the complexities of mental health conditions. AI can help foster collaborations between mental health professionals, AI researchers, data scientists, and policymakers to constantly improve and refine AI applications in mental health care. Stakeholders can allocate resources and funding for research initiatives exploring the intersection of AI and mental health. Through digital platforms, information, educational content, and resources can be disseminated globally, contributing to increased awareness, education, and empowerment.

Reducing Stigma and Increasing Awareness: While many illness conditions carry stigma, like in HIV or cancer, none parallels the stigma associated with mental illnesses. Stigma regarding mental health issues has been a major concern for health seekers creating a barrier in treatment as well as rehabilitation of individuals with mental illness. Owing to stigma and the fear of their identity being associated with mental health issues, many individuals hesitate to bring forth their concerns leading to further worsening of their symptoms; and by the time they consult a professional, symptoms aggravate or become chronic. AI has a big implication here, as individuals may feel comfortable discussing their emotions with an AI-based virtual assistant or chatbot maintaining their anonymity as there is no fear of judgement or stigma. This can encourage individuals to seek help earlier, improving overall mental health outcomes.

The online communities and social media platforms provide spaces for individuals to share experiences, find support, and access information anonymously, reducing stigma and fostering a sense of community. Similarly educational platforms facilitate the dissemination of accurate information about mental health, empowering individuals to recognize symptoms and seek help in early stages.

The Challenges

Despite the promises and avenues, ensuring fair and equal access to technological advancements of AI and integrating it with mental health is not an easy task. Factors like infrastructure limitations, digital literacy, and disparities in resources need to be addressed to ensure that the benefits of AI reach everyone, regardless of location or socioeconomic status.

While AI offers immense potential, ethical considerations such as data privacy, bias in algorithms, and equitable access to these innovations need to be addressed. Ensuring ethical use of AI in mental health and addressing concerns about data privacy and biases in algorithms remains crucial for its successful implementation. Overall, the fusion of AI techniques and mental health care holds great potential for improving access, efficiency, and effectiveness in supporting mental well-being.

AI tools are here to complement human expertise and are not a replacement for human interaction or expertise. Ensuring privacy, maintaining ethical standards, and continuously improving AI systems are crucial to maximizing the positive impact on mental health while minimizing potential risks.

As we figure out the promising possibilities of convergence of AI with mental health, the proposed developments come with their own unique challenges.

Whether any AI system will have universal approach and acceptability: We humans always have taken an underlying pride over the complexities of the human mind or the psyche, and that every human is different from the other. This gives an apprehension whether AI would be capable of understanding the complex processes of the ill human mind with algorithms. Also, whether an AI programme developed for a particular population will be effective for similar populations in other parts of the world.

Whether it will be equally effective in conditions other than psychosis, developmental disabilities, depression and anxiety: While certain mental health conditions have a more or less uniform pattern of manifestation, there are several other conditions, where person A and person B suffering from the same diagnosed illness may have slightly different sets of symptoms. Whether AI will ever have that amount of data which can cover all the possibilities, will be a key factor for success.

How AI will tackle comorbidity issues in Mental health: Comorbidity is a rule rather than exception in Psychiatry. As AI will attempt to filter out information to get a direction towards diagnoses, numerous possibilities of comorbidity will be confusing for the algorithm.

Whether AI will be intelligent enough to grasp the concept of normality and abnormality: With progressing days, the concept of normality and abnormality is shifting. Subjective and objective differences in the opinion about normalcy of the mental state of an individual often differs. In this scenario, AI systems may give confounding results. AI may also have a tough time looking into issues coming out of novelty-seeking behaviour, or symptoms which are below diagnostic threshold and other behaviour which might look problematic objectively but not subjectively.

Whether AI will be intelligent enough to understand sarcasm in human communication: This is already a known challenge for AI. Human language and communication often do not follow simple rules, and words mean something different than what is spoken. In this scenario, profiling or filtering data based on standard rules may give erroneous results.

As the scope of integration of AI and mental health grows gradually, new frontiers open that suggests the following:

Evaluation and Feedback Loop: Regularly assess the effectiveness of AI interventions in mental health through rigorous evaluation methods. Use feedback from both patients and mental health professionals to iterate and improve AI-based tools and services.

Continuously monitor AI systems to prevent biases and ensure fair and accurate assessments.

Integration with Existing Healthcare Systems: Ensure seamless integration of AI tools into existing healthcare systems, making them accessible and user-friendly for both patients and practitioners.

For Continuous Development and Adaptation, stay updated with technological advancements and continuously adapt AI algorithms and models to enhance their accuracy, reliability, and relevance in addressing mental health challenges. By fostering a symbiotic relationship between AI and mental health, we can create a more efficient, accessible, and personalized mental healthcare system, ultimately reducing the burden of mental health disorders on individuals and society.

References

Castillo-Sánchez, G., Marques, G., Dorronzoro, E., et al. (2020). Suicide risk assessment using machine learning and social networks: A scoping review. *Journal of Medical Systems, 44*(205), 1. https://doi.org/10.1007/s10916-020-01669-5

Hirani, R., Noruzi, K., Khuram, H., Hussaini, A. S., Aifuwa, E. I., Ely, K. E., Lewis, J. M., Gabr, A. E., Smiley, A., Tiwari, R. K., & Etienne, M. (2024). Artificial intelligence and healthcare: A journey through history, present innovations, and future possibilities. *Life (Basel, Switzerland), 14*(5), 557. https://doi.org/10.3390/life14050557

Lewanowicz, A., Wiśniewski, M., & Oronowicz-Jaśkowiak, W. (2022). The use of machine learning to support the therapeutic process - strengths and weaknesses. *Postepy Psychiatrii Neurologii, 31*(4), 167–173. https://doi.org/10.5114/ppn.2022.125050

Linthicum, K. P., Schafer, K. M., & Ribeiro, J. D. (2019). Machine learning in suicide science: Applications and ethics. *Behavioral Sciences & the Law, 37*(3), 214–222. https://doi.org/10.1002/bsl.2392

Ryu, S., Lee, H., Lee, D. K., Kim, S. W., & Kim, C. E. (2019). Detection of Suicide Attempters among Suicide Ideators Using Machine Learning. *Psychiatry Investigation, 16*(8), 588–593. https://doi.org/10.30773/pi.2019.06.19

Chapter 4
AI in the Detection of Mental Health Problems

Abstract As we discussed in previous chapters about the general scope of integrating AI in mental health, we move further on specific domains on how AI can be of specific use in mental health services. This chapter focuses on the transformative impact of AI for screening mental ill health conditions, diagnosis as well as prognosis. We explore how large datasets are analysed using machine learning techniques, natural language processing, and predictive analytics to reveal trends and risk factors related to mental health issues. It emphasizes the potential of AI technologies to increase the speed and accuracy of mental health assessments through an extensive analysis of recent research and discusses future prospects, obstacles, and ethical issues related to the smooth integration of AI into clinical practice.

Keywords Mental health screening · Diagnosis · Prognosis · Risk assessment

Use and Impact of AI in Mental Health Screening, Diagnosis, and Prognosis

There is a growing need for creative and effective ways to improve early detection in mental health by screening, increasing accuracy in diagnosis and better prediction of prognosis of the various problems to prevent the occurrences as the prevalence of mental health issues rises worldwide.

We have discussed the human tendency to have apprehensions when it comes to our health. We always prefer to consult the best possible doctor when we have a major health issue and do not hesitate to take a second opinion. So why should we turn to machines or software when there is an expert doctor around. Particularly in Asian or Indian context, expert physicians are revered and usually get respect from people. So are the machines capable enough like the expert doctors or the professionals.

A part of the answer to these questions lies in the following data regarding prevalence of mental ill health conditions and availability of health infrastructure and resources. Contrary to the general perception, mental health conditions are more prevalent and showing an ever-increasing trend. As per the Global Burden of Disease

S. Halder et al., *Navigating AI in Mental Health Care*,
https://doi.org/10.1007/978-981-96-9744-1_4

(GBD) study, 970 million people or 1 in every 8 people, around the world were living with a mental disorder in the year 2019. Among these anxiety and depressive disorders were the most common. The graver conditions like schizophrenia though were lesser percentage wise; there is a stable increase in its numbers (approx.24 million globally in 2019) and related disability (Solmi et al., 2023). Global surveys in different countries might give some slightly different, but more or less similar figures. After the COVID-19 pandemic, there has been a sharp spike in reporting of mental health issues globally. Researchers suggest that the pandemic might have triggered mental health issues among the vulnerable and relapse or worsening of existing mental health symptoms. In 2020, the number of people living with anxiety and depressive disorders rose significantly because of the COVID-19 pandemic, with initial estimates showing a 26% and 28% increase respectively for anxiety and major depressive disorders in just one year (WHO, 2022). There were also increasing reports of self- injurious behaviour and completed suicide during the COVID-19 pandemic. The trend is the same for all mental health conditions, be it for children, adolescents, adults, or the ageing population. All these point towards the global need of catering to ever increasing mental health needs of the population. However, the resources in terms of trained professionals as well as infrastructure to meet this demand has mostly been disproportionate in most, if not in all countries. The World Health Organization (2021) mentions that health systems have not yet adequately responded to the needs of people with mental disorders and are significantly under-resourced. There is a wide gap between the need for treatment and its provision worldwide and is often poor in quality when delivered. For example, only 29% of people with psychosis and only one third of people with depression receive formal mental health care (Moitra et al., 2022). There is also a pattern of skewed distribution of professionals, where urban centres usually have a crowding of professionals, while rural or semiurban areas lack adequate number of trained people, resulting in crowding at most of the urban centres, keeping urban mental health services overstretched and burdened. While every country strives and efforts to keep up with the demands of its population's healthcare needs, the process of training healthcare professionals, including mental health professionals is a task which takes a considerable period of time, excluding the period of super specialization. By the time a professional is ready, an unevenly matched number of clinical populations also happens to increase manyfold. In such a scenario, it is often advised to create a pool of health workers who can be given a basic training to work at preliminary level to identify and give appropriate recommendations to clients. But there are always apprehensions regarding the clinical judgement in absence of full-fledged professional training. Psychiatry is one filed of medicine which often comes under radar for the approach it takes to diagnose its clients. There is often certain level of subjectivity in clinical judgement of professionals in diagnosing and to no surprise two trained professional might differ on the diagnosis and therapeutic approach they deem appropriate for a same client. This is an ideal situation where AI can be of good assistance to help professionals in making better clinical judgement, be it a trained professionals or semi trained health workers. In both cases AI could be handy to ease the workload assisting in the diagnostic screening, diagnosis, and overall therapy process of the client.

We also need to understand the process of screening and diagnosis in mental health services, as mental health is one field of medicine which typically does not have laboratory-based diagnostic test. Unlike other field of medicine, where a blood test or a CT scan or x ray can provide valuable diagnostic information; they are of little use in mental health related diagnostic process. There are psychological tests of different kinds though, which help in quantifying the severity of the symptoms, categorizing them, giving an indication of underlying pathology or personality construct which helps in validating or support the diagnosis made by the professional. Certain types of psychological tests or rating scale do help in screening specific disorders, despite that an in-depth clinical history, a mental status examination is must for making a clinical diagnosis. We take a further look at these concepts to understand the compatibility of AI in the existing procedure of diagnosing and screening in mental health.

The process of Diagnosing in Mental health: Assigning a diagnosis for mental health conditions essentially depends on someone meeting the criteria specified in the classificatory system, like the Diagnostic and Statistical manual (DSM) or the International Classification of Disease (ICD). This may appear simple as ticking a list, but to ascertain whether an individual meet the criteria for a clinical diagnosis, a thorough assessment is done by trained and licensed professionals, such as clinical psychologists, psychiatrist, or a psychiatric social worker. As mentioned earlier, the process typically involves taking clinical history from the client as well as informants or caregivers. Lapses and inconsistency in this part of the process are very much expected, making the task challenging for the professional. There might be differences in reporting of symptom from the client and care givers perspective. Further, a mental status examination (MSE) of the client is done. The MSE can be understood as a semi structured interview, where in the behavioural observation of the client as well as responses to specific questions by the client gives an idea of his cognitive functions, thought process as well as psychopathology at that point of time. At this stage also certain clients may not be very cooperative or elaborate depending on their insight and symptom severity. The professionals filter the relevant information, and using clinical judgement make a diagnostic formulation for a client. This formulation gives way to a diagnosis as per the classificatory systems. However, despite all professional training there is possibility of error owing to different reasons including insufficient information or non-cooperation from clients to name a few. To support or validate their clinical impression or the diagnosis, psychological assessments are often done by trained clinical professionals.

Now talking about Screening: It may appear that the process of screening is uniform and mandatory for all mental health conditions. However, screening is more implied in conditions where clients are doubted to have confounding symptoms and need to be ruled out, or they need to be assessed if the symptoms are severe enough to be clinically diagnosed. Screening, thus, is an initial step to identify individuals who might be at risk or showing signs of a particular mental health issue. It involves using tools like questionnaires, or observations to detect potential problems. Thus, screening is handy to identify potential cases at risk of developing major mental health issues. Screening doesn't offer a definitive diagnosis rather indicates whether further evaluation is necessary. Screening procedures are also very helpful in community and primary care settings, or at places lacking adequately trained manpower. A proper screening can help deciding the course of action for referral primary care to higher centre for advanced consultation. It may be noted that the process of screening is not much required if clinical symptoms are very florid and not marred with comorbid condition. The process of screening may not be full proof and at times may give confounding results owing to different factors like poor comprehension capability and educational background of the client, cultural differences in presentation of symptoms, subjective distress, and false reporting. In above scenario, there is ample scope of use of AI in the process, which can aid professionals in making better diagnostic impression of their clients.

Once a potential issue is identified through screening, diagnosis comes into play. Mental health professionals, such as psychologists or psychiatrists, conduct a thorough assessment. They evaluate symptoms, history, and sometimes use standardized criteria (like those in the Diagnostic and Statistical Manual of Mental Disorders, DSM) to establish a formal diagnosis. This step helps to categorize and understand the specific mental health condition an individual might be experiencing. Once a potential issue is identified through screening, diagnosis comes into play. Mental health professionals, such as psychologists or psychiatrists, conduct a thorough assessment. They evaluate symptoms, history, and sometimes use standardized criteria (like those in the Diagnostic and Statistical Manual of Mental Disorders, DSM) to establish a formal diagnosis. This step helps to categorize and understand the specific mental health condition an individual might be experiencing.

What is Screening, Diagnosis, and Prognosis

In mental health, screening, diagnosis, and prognosis play crucial roles in understanding, assessing, and predicting the course of various mental health conditions. Thus, it's good to understand these terms.

Prognosis: *The APA defines prognosis as a prediction of the course, duration, severity, and outcome of a condition, disease, or disorder. Prognosis may be given before any treatment is undertaken, so that the patient or client can weigh the benefits of different treatment options.* Assessing the likely course and outcome of a mental health condition helps in setting realistic expectations for patients and their families. It guides mental health professionals in providing appropriate support, therapy, and resources needed for recovery. Thus, prognosis involves predicting the likely course and outcome of a mental health condition. It considers various factors, such as the nature and severity of the disorder, the individual's response to treatment, any coexisting conditions, and external influences like social support. Prognosis isn't always straightforward as it can vary greatly among individuals with the same diagnosis. It helps in guiding treatment planning and managing expectations regarding recovery or management of symptoms. Each of these components is essential in providing appropriate care and support for individuals dealing with mental health issues. They collectively inform the development of treatment plans tailored to the specific needs of the individual. Regular reassessment may occur to track progress, adjust treatment approaches, and update prognostic expectations.

The conventional method of predicting prognosis has often been criticized by many experts, mostly on the grounds that it gives a pessimistic overview of chances of recovery for patients with chronic illness or with severe level of symptoms or poor psychosocial support. While these factors are vital in recovery, but a quantified poor prognosis may influence the treating team losing hope on the particular client, and risk of sense of indifference towards them, particularly those in inpatient care. However, despite the prognosis, every client has the right of being treated with same optimism. One of the important relevance of predicting prognosis is that it also delves on probable course of development of symptoms or relapse of the client. In mental health, much of this prognostic prediction lies in the clinical expertise of the trained professionals, who may not be very accurate in weighing all the factors involved. In this scenario, AI can be of much help in assisting in making better prediction regarding the prognosis and treatment outcome.

Screening: Early identification of mental health issues through screening allows for timely intervention. Detecting symptoms or risk factors at an early stage can prevent the escalation of conditions, improving the chances of successful treatment.

Diagnosis: Accurate diagnosis is crucial for understanding the specific mental health disorder a person is experiencing. It helps in tailoring the treatment plan according to the individual's needs. Misdiagnosis or delayed diagnosis can lead to ineffective treatments or unnecessary suffering. Each mental health condition is unique, and an accurate diagnosis enables healthcare providers to offer targeted and personalized care. It ensures that the treatment plan addresses the specific symptoms and underlying causes of the individual's mental health issue.

Reducing Stigma and Misconceptions by Education and Awareness: Through screening, diagnosis, and prognosis, there is an opportunity to educate individuals about mental health. This can help reduce stigma, increase awareness, and encourage people to seek help without fear of judgement.

Other Implications

Data Collection and Research: Screening and diagnosis contribute valuable data for Public Health research and policymaking. Understanding the prevalence, patterns, and outcomes of mental health conditions aids in developing better strategies for prevention, intervention, and support at a societal level.

Overall Well-being-like Quality of Life: Timely screening and accurate diagnosis lead to appropriate treatment, which significantly improves a person's quality of life. It can enhance their ability to function in daily activities, maintain relationships, and contribute positively to their community.

Prevention of Escalation: Preventive Measures: Early identification and intervention can prevent mild issues from developing into severe or chronic mental health conditions. It allows for the implementation of preventive measures and lifestyle changes that may mitigate the progression of certain disorders.

In essence, screening, diagnosis, and prognosis are essential components in mental health care. They enable early identification, personalized treatment, and better outcomes for individuals, thereby positively impacting both the individual and society as a whole. There is a growing need for creative and effective ways to improve early detection by screening, increasing accuracy in diagnosis and better prediction of prognosis of the various problem to prevent the occurrences as the prevalence of mental health issues rises worldwide.

How AI is Being Used in Screening of Mental Health Conditions

AI in screening for mental health issues has been revolutionary due to its ability to analyse vast amounts of data and detect patterns that might not be apparent to humans. Through various methods like Natural Language Processing (NLP), machine learning, deep learning, and predictive analytics, AI systems can be used to analyse text and speech, for behavioural cues to identify potential signs of mental health conditions.

One significant advantage is the scalability of AI-driven screening. These systems can handle a large volume of individuals' data and patterns efficiently, providing a preliminary assessment and flagging cases that might require further attention from mental health professionals. This scalability is crucial, especially in scenarios where there's a shortage of mental health practitioners or when accessibility to mental health services is limited.

Moreover, AI-driven screening tools can operate 24/7 through programming and automation, allowing individuals to seek help or intervention at any time, reducing the wait time for assessments and potentially preventing crises by offering timely support. This accessibility encourages individuals who might otherwise hesitate to seek help due to stigma or other barriers.

However, there are notable challenges and ethical considerations. Privacy and data security are crucial, especially when dealing with sensitive mental health information. Ensuring that these AI systems comply with strict ethical standards, maintain confidentiality, and protect user data is essential to gain trust and encourage people to use these tools.

Additionally, while AI can assist in screening, it cannot replace the human aspect of mental health care. AI should complement, not substitute, the expertise and empathy of trained professionals. Hence, it's vital to integrate these tools into a broader mental healthcare framework, allowing professionals to use the insights provided by AI as a part of their diagnostic and treatment processes.

Continuous improvement and validation of these AI systems are necessary to enhance accuracy and effectiveness. Collaborations between mental health experts and AI developers are essential to refine these tools, ensuring they are culturally sensitive, unbiased, and effective across diverse populations.

In summary, the use of AI in screening for mental health problems has the potential to significantly improve early detection, accessibility, and overall mental health care. However, responsible implementation, ethical considerations, and a collaborative approach are critical to maximizing its benefits while addressing its limitations.

Accuracy in Diagnosis

The use of AI in the accuracy of diagnosing mental health problems has shown promising potential. AI applications, particularly machine learning algorithms, are being employed to aid mental health professionals in several ways:

Pattern Recognition: AI algorithms can analyse vast amounts of data from various sources, including patient interviews, medical records, and even social media, to recognize patterns that might indicate certain mental health conditions. These patterns might be subtle and complex, making them difficult for humans to identify but easier for AI systems to detect.

Early Detection: AI can help in the early detection of mental health issues by identifying risk factors and warning signs that might go unnoticed by individuals or even healthcare providers. Early detection allows for earlier intervention, potentially preventing the exacerbation of conditions.

Personalized Treatment: By analysing data from a large number of cases, AI can assist in recommending personalized treatment plans. It can consider factors like the patient's history, genetic predispositions, responses to different treatments, and lifestyle choices to suggest more tailored and effective interventions.

Reducing Bias: AI systems can help mitigate biases in diagnosis that might arise due to human subjectivity or lack of diverse experiences. These systems can process information objectively, potentially leading to more accurate and fairer diagnoses across different demographics. However, caution should be exercised to ensure that the data used by AI for the analyses should not be biased.

Improving Efficiency: AI tools can significantly speed up the diagnostic process. They can analyse large volumes of data quickly, providing healthcare professionals with insights and recommendations promptly, thereby enhancing the efficiency of mental health services.

However, there are **challenges and considerations** in the use of AI in mental health diagnosis:

Data Privacy and Ethics: Utilizing personal data for AI analysis raises concerns about privacy and ethical considerations. Protecting patient confidentiality and ensuring data security is crucial in the development and deployment of AI systems in mental health. Data and privacy regulations for various countries should also be adhered to when dealing with patient data.

Reliability and Validation: AI algorithms need extensive validation to ensure their reliability and accuracy. The quality and diversity of the data used to train these algorithms significantly impact their effectiveness. Biases within datasets can lead to skewed or incorrect conclusions.

Supplementing, Not Replacing Human Expertise: AI should be seen as a tool to support mental health professionals rather than replace them. Human judgement, empathy, and contextual understanding remain irreplaceable in the field of mental health care.

In conclusion, while AI shows immense potential in improving the accuracy of diagnosing mental health problems, its successful implementation requires careful consideration of ethical, privacy, and reliability concerns. When integrated thoughtfully into mental health practices, AI can complement and enhance the capabilities of healthcare professionals, leading to more accurate diagnoses and better treatment outcomes for patients.

Better Prediction of Prognosis:

AI has shown promising potential in enhancing the prediction of prognosis for mental health issues. Here's an elaboration on this point:

Data Analysis and Pattern Recognition: AI systems excel at analysing vast amounts of data. In mental health, these systems can sift through extensive patient records, genetic information, brain imaging data, and even social media activity to identify patterns that might correlate with particular mental health outcomes. By recognizing these patterns, AI can help predict the progression of mental health conditions.

Early Detection and Intervention: Machine learning algorithms can be trained to detect subtle changes or early signs of mental health issues that might not be immediately apparent to human clinicians. For instance, by analysing speech patterns, facial expressions, or even keystroke dynamics, AI models can potentially identify signs of depression, anxiety, or other disorders before they manifest overtly. Early detection allows for timely intervention, preventing the exacerbation of conditions.

Personalized Treatment Plans: AI can assist in creating personalized treatment plans by considering an individual's unique data, including their genetic makeup, lifestyle, environmental factors, and treatment response history. By analysing this data, AI systems can suggest tailored interventions or medication regimes that are more likely to be effective for a particular patient, improving prognosis and treatment outcomes.

Risk Assessment and Prevention: AI-driven models can assess an individual's risk of developing certain mental health disorders based on their biological, behavioural, and environmental factors. By identifying high-risk individuals, preventive measures or interventions can be implemented, potentially reducing the likelihood or severity of mental health problems.

Continuous Monitoring and Feedback: Wearable devices and smartphone apps integrated with AI can continuously monitor an individual's mental health indicators. These systems can provide real-time feedback, suggesting coping mechanisms or alerting healthcare providers or family members if concerning changes are detected, thus allowing for timely interventions and support.

Reducing Bias and Improving Accuracy: AI models can mitigate biases that might exist in traditional diagnostic processes. By relying on objective data analysis, AI can provide more accurate and consistent prognostic assessments, minimizing human errors and subjective judgements.

Research and Development: AI helps in accelerating mental health research by analysing vast datasets from clinical trials, studies, and patient records. This aids in understanding the underlying mechanisms of mental disorders, leading to the development of more effective treatments and interventions.

While AI can significantly aid in prognosis prediction, it should complement, not replace, the expertise and empathy of mental health professionals in providing comprehensive care.

What are the Risks: In midst of all the positive hopes AI brings in the domain, we must also be aware of the potential risks of using AI in screening and diagnosis procedures. It's true that every technology has its own loopholes and limitations, but AI probably is meeting fiercest of criticism as well as apprehensions about possible unwanted effects and harm it may cause for its users. While illnesses and health conditions carry their own stigma, the stigma associated with mental health conditions probably is unparalleled.

Developers are thus apprehensive, that how the general mass would adapt to it. The fear of use and misuse of data will be a big challenge to counter.

Universal application? One of the major challenges which AI appear to face when applied in mental health is regarding its universal application. Mental health is a very versatile domain, and its presentation and manifestation vary across the globe. Despite having diagnostic criteria, cultural factors do influence the symptoms in a client. In such a scenario, whether an AI algorithm developed on a database of a specific population will be good enough to deliver in other parts of the globe is a big question.

References

Solmi, M., Seitidis, G., Mavridis, D., et al. (2023). Incidence, prevalence, and global burden of schizophrenia - data, with critical appraisal, from the Global Burden of Disease (GBD) 2019. *Molecular Psychiatry.* https://doi.org/10.1038/s41380-023-02138-4

World Health Organization. (2021). *Mental health atlas 2020.* World Health Organization.

World Health Organization. (2022). *Mental health and COVID-19: Early evidence of the pandemic's impact.* World Health Organization.

Moitra, M., Santomauro, D., Collins, P. Y., Vos, T., Whiteford, H., Saxena, S., et al. (2022). The global gap in treatment coverage for major depressive disorder in 84 countries from 2000–2019: A systematic review and Bayesian meta-regression analysis. *PLOS Medicine, 19*(2), Article e1003901. https://doi.org/10.1371/journal.pmed.1003901

Part II
Use of AI to Better Decode Mental Health Conditions

Chapter 5
Anxiety Spectrum Disorders

Abstract Anxiety spectrum disorders are among the most common mental health issues worldwide, affecting millions of individuals and significantly impacting their daily lives. Traditional approaches to diagnosing and treating anxiety, while effective, often face challenges related to accessibility, cost, and personalized care. In recent years, Artificial Intelligence (AI) has emerged as a promising tool in mental health care, offering innovative solutions for the diagnosis, treatment, and management of anxiety spectrum disorders. This chapter explores the role of AI in addressing anxiety spectrum disorders, covering the various applications, benefits, limitations, and future directions of AI in this field.

Keywords Anxiety spectrum disorder · Early detection · Prediction · AI-based intervention

A Brief About Anxiety Spectrum Disorders

Anxiety spectrum disorders encompass a range of conditions characterized by excessive worry, fear, and related behavioural disturbances. The common types of anxiety disorders include (not exhaustive):

- Generalized Anxiety Disorder (GAD): Characterized by persistent and excessive worry about various aspects of life.
- Panic Disorder: Characterized by recurrent and unexpected panic attacks, accompanied by physical symptoms like heart palpitations and shortness of breath.
- Social Anxiety Disorder (SAD): Characterized by intense fear of social situations and being judged or scrutinized by others.
- Specific Phobias: Characterized by irrational fears of specific objects or situations, such as heights, animals, or flying.
- Obsessive–Compulsive Disorder (OCD): Characterized by recurrent, unwanted thoughts (obsessions), and repetitive behaviours (compulsions).
- Post-Traumatic Stress Disorder (PTSD): Characterized by anxiety triggered by traumatic events, leading to flashbacks, nightmares, and severe anxiety.

S. Halder et al., *Navigating AI in Mental Health Care*,
https://doi.org/10.1007/978-981-96-9744-1_5

There are several other categories listed in the classificatory systems, both DSM and the ICD, but the above more or less present the gamut of anxiety spectrum disorders.

How Prevalent Anxiety Disorders Are?

Anxiety disorders represent the most common category of mental illnesses affecting millions of individuals worldwide and imposing significant burdens on both those affected and society at large. They are prevalent across all age groups, genders, and cultures significantly impairing an individual's ability to function in daily life, affecting their personal, social, and professional relationships. The global burden of anxiety disorders highlights the need for effective and accessible interventions. Any anxiety disorder has an approximate lifetime prevalence of 16% and an approximate 12-month prevalence of 11% (Carter et al., 2001; Wittchen et al., 1994). In general, the incidence of anxiety disorders varies greatly as per research, with estimates of a larger prevalence in rich Western nations compared to developing nations. Anxiety disorders were the most common mental disorders in the recent national epidemiological research conducted in China, with a lifetime prevalence of 7.6% and an annual prevalence of 5.0% (Chang et al., 2021). These illnesses will cause a considerable increase in the disease burden.

However, a major issue with anxiety disorders is that most individuals with anxiety disorders, when in subclinical or even mild severity, are capable of continuing functioning in their daily lives though with some amount of impairment. A majority of them do not deem appropriate for a professional consultation and seek it only when the symptoms become disabling for them. Thus, the real prevalence of anxiety disorders might be larger than reported in the surveys.

Screening, Early Detection, and Diagnosis of Anxiety Spectrum Disorders & Role of AI

Management of anxiety spectrum disorders essentially includes the basic processes of screening and diagnosing, which is uniform for other disorders too.

An individual consulting for anxiety issues will report his problems as per his distress associated with the symptoms, without any insight about diagnostic criteria of the ICD or the DSM. Some may also have certain attention seeking issues and may exaggerate their symptoms and might provide irrelevant details too. It is the expertise of the professional to filter relevant information and arrange them in sequence as per the progression of the illness, which transpires in the form of clinical history. We reiterate that, even though this process is same for any other mental ill health condition, the precipitating factors or stressors are different for all and will provide

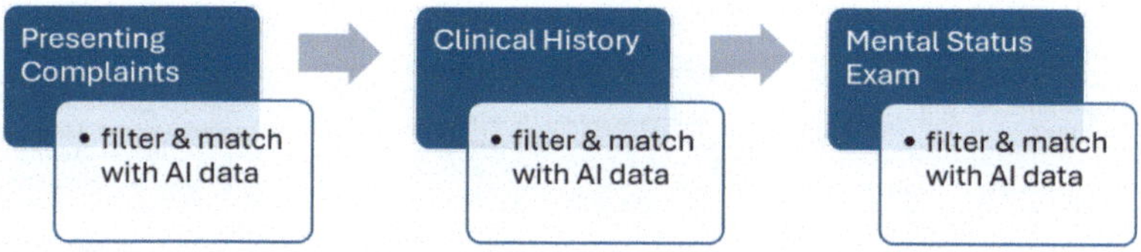

Fig. 5.1 AI assisted clinical interview and diagnostic process

vital clues, how individuals are similar or differ to react under similar circumstances. The process further involves gathering crucial information regarding a patient's past history, any family history of anxiety disorder or any other mental ill health condition, the psychosocial environment of the patient, development pattern since childhood, functioning as well as premorbid personality pattern. A human mental health professional while eliciting and filtering these information fits them into existing theoretical models providing a justification of the diagnosis. For a change if we think this process to be assisted by AI, the process will remain the same; however, the information from individual patients will be treated like data and add to decision-making with statistical level of difference (Fig. 5.1).

Further, the patient is engaged in a process called mental status examination. The mental status examination is a structured assessment of the patient's behavioural and cognitive functioning, which includes descriptions of the patient's appearance and general behaviour, level of consciousness and attentiveness, motor and speech activity, mood and affect, thought and perception, attitude and insight, the reaction evoked in the examiner, and, finally, higher cognitive abilities (Martin, 1990). It is important to note that even though these processes look distinct, done in different phases following a sequence and separate from each other, they are essentially entwined with each other. The information in each of these phases or stages must corroborate and supplement each other, and discrepancies if any, which are not rare, warrants a careful look by the expert professional.

Though not always necessary, psychological assessment tools further provide an idea about the presence or absence of any specific pathology or symptoms as well as severity of the symptoms.

How AI Can Be Integrated in the Same Process

We will discuss this through a case study. Mr J is a 38-year-old male, an information technology professional, working in the marketing wing of a multinational company. He presented with complaints of feeling stressed, anxious, and restless most of the time, constant worries, disturbed sleep, palpitations, sweating, and occasional episodes of panic for the past 3 years. The symptoms had a gradual onset without any significant precipitating factor and are continuous in nature with fluctuating progress. He never had any treatment before and reported was very anxious in nature and died

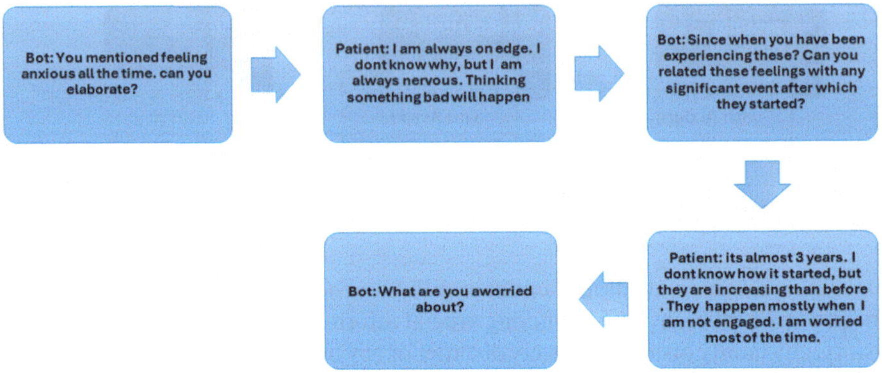

Fig. 5.2 Sample elicitation of responses by chatbot

of cardiac arrest. He was diagnosed with generalized anxiety disorder. Eliciting the exact nature of complaints in this case is important to establish the sequence of development of symptoms, whether they developed simultaneously or in different phases. As many symptoms of generalized anxiety and panic are overlapping, it is vital to establish which set of symptoms is predominant for most appropriate diagnosis. While mental health professionals are trained for this, the task may be monotonous or tiring at times. Thus, the task, when assigned to an AI program, can nicely elicit the same set of responses and categorize them to appropriate categories, while ruling out other conditions (Fig. 5.2).

A sample conversation between a professional and client will look like the statements above. An AI-based chatbot can also elicit the same responses; however, the chatbot will pick the clues from specific words used like, *"always on edge", "nervous", and "something bad will happen*". There will be further possibilities of ruling out differential conditions by asking related questions, which even human professionals do, but as mentioned earlier, it could be a monotonous and tiring task. The AI programme may possibly combine data input from different modalities including text or speech of the patient, facial expressions, psychomotor movements through camera feed to provide assistance in decision-making for the human mental health professional.

Clinical history is often said to be the most vital tool for diagnosis in mental health. However, gathering reliable and adequate information from patients could be tricky, as patients with anxiety disorder could be over detailing. Similarly, when taking the mental status examination of the patient, the queries from an AI chatbot will always be structured as per the designed algorithm, and they have better chances of being consistent to elicit specific information. Every piece of information not only aids in the diagnosis of the patient but will also add to the existing dataset for better data analysis.

Further talking about assessments, there are a host of rating scales which are used for assessing the presence, nature as well as severity of the anxiety and related symptoms. The most commonly used scales (not exhaustive) include the Hamilton

Anxiety Rating scale, Beck Anxiety Inventory, of which the former is clinician rated and the later, self-rated by the patient. While computerized versions of rating scales are available nowadays for easy scoring and documentation, there is much scope of integrating AI in this process. The impression from these rating scales though are not always conclusive and diagnostic, as they are reported to have limitation in differentiating between anxiety and depression in a primary care population (Muntingh et al., 2011), or poor ability to discriminate between anxiolytic and antidepressant effects, and somatic anxiety versus somatic side effects (Maier et al., 1988). In such a scenario, the rating scores can be corroborated by an AI-based tool for a better informed decision.

Challenges in Diagnosing of Anxiety Disorder Using Artificial Intelligence

Mental ill health conditions are often overlapping in nature to the extent that comorbidity is said to be the rule rather than exception. Despite specific diagnostic guidelines, anxiety spectrum disorders could be challenging to diagnose. Not all conditions are severe enough to be detected by naked eyes, and demand expertise. Symptoms might be at sub clinical level yet be disabling in nature. New mental health issues are emerging at the same time corresponding to modern societal and psychosocial environmental changes. A persistent and severely incapacitating illness, anxiety disorder manifests itself in a variety of clinical ways. Worldwide prevalence, according to epidemiological studies, is 5%, while 10% of people have subclinical symptoms. Remarkably, 9% of teenagers have clinical characteristics. Thus, a larger number of individuals are at probability of being misdiagnosed. Predicting anxiety disorder using a machine learning algorithm analysis model is hence highly significant.

One vital aspect of anxiety spectrum disorders is that there is an evident set psychophysiological response in certain conditions, especially generalized anxiety disorder, panic disorder, and phobia. Invariably there is also a certain level of disruptions in sleep pattern, perspiration levels, breathing pattern as well as muscle tone in these conditions which are objectively visible and can also be easily quantified and recorded through appropriate measurement tools.

In this context, AI-based programmes can analyse behavioural/ physiological data from wearable devices and smartphones, such as sleep patterns, physical activity, and social interactions, to identify signs of anxiety aiding in diagnosis. The advantage of these devices is that they can provide accurate data from the past too, minimising error in personal reporting.

For example, we look at sample talk between therapist and a client, presented primarily with symptoms of panic.

Therapist: So... Can you elaborate on your concerns?

Patient: I feel panicky.

Therapist: Can you help me understand, how does it feel to you?

Patient: It's very intense, I feel like I am going to die.

Therapist: Okay... you feel like you are going to die. When does this happen, and how frequent it is?

Patient: Not sure, it may happen any time of the day.

Therapist: And how frequent is it?

Patient: Not sure, it happens irregularly. Maybe twice or thrice a week, maybe daily.

Therapist: Okay... and how long do they last? Have you noticed them happening more in certain conditions or certain places?

Patient: five to ten minutes, may be longer. Am always anxious. It can happen anywhere.

Upon enquiry she was unable to give satisfactory details regarding duration of the panic attacks, its likely triggers, mentioning they could happen anytime or any place.

In cases like these, wearable devices can provide valuable assistance in tracking incidents of significant variation in psychophysiological responses that are indicative of panic, giving an accurate measurement of the incident, which can be verified with the patient. In this context, it is worthy to mention Woebot, an AI chatbot, which uses NLP to engage users in conversations and screen for anxiety symptoms (Brown, 2021). It asks users questions about their triggers, onset time, associated thoughts, and behaviours, providing real-time feedback and recommendations based on their responses. Other AI-Driven Diagnostic Platforms such as Quartet Health, use machine learning algorithms to analyse patient data and provide clinicians with insights and recommendations for diagnosing and treating anxiety disorders. These platforms integrate data from electronic health records, patient surveys, and clinical assessments to offer a comprehensive view of the patient's mental health.

Using Artificial Intelligence in Counselling and Psychotherapy for Anxiety Disorders

Evidence-based research indicates that the combination of psychotherapy and pharmacotherapy is much more useful than medication alone for treating anxiety disorders. As such, psychotherapy can be utilized in clinical practice to treat anxiety disorders alone or to maximize the impact of medical treatment. According to various national guidelines, psychotherapy—such as cognitive-behavioural therapy, relaxation therapy, systematic desensitization, exposure–response prevention, and other psychotherapies—should be used as the initial line of treatment for anxiety disorders. While the primary focus of counselling and psychotherapy is impacted by a variety of treatments, they are all aimed at helping clients change their dysfunctional beliefs and thoughts to improve their behaviour. Most of these methods locate a problematic behaviour and change it for a better or more constructive one. Conventionally, counselling and psychotherapy have been done engaging the therapist and the client in a one-to-one session. But to provide any of these interventions, licensed therapists with professional training are needed. However, there aren't enough of these therapists, particularly in rural or undeveloped areas many patients don't have access to standardized, effective care. As a matter of fact, a very small percentage of patients who have undergone psychotherapy received formal psychotherapy.

Artificial Intelligence (AI)-assisted psychotherapy provides an alternative to traditional face-to-face psychotherapy in the absence of such services. The treatment of anxiety disorders and other disorders can be significantly improved using Internet Cognitive-Behavioural Therapy (iCBT) and Computerized Cognitive-Behavioural Therapy (cCBT), according to several meta-analyses. Woebot, a completely automated conversational assistant, can help patients recognize their feelings and learn coping mechanisms to lessen anxiety and symptoms. However, these technologies are not a replacement for human therapists, and research suggests their efficacy is better compared to self-help behavioural intervention (Eltahawy et al., 2024).

Personalized Treatment Plans and Tailored Interventions: Despite the availability of evidence-based psychotherapeutic and pharmacological treatments, the reality is that not all patients experience the same level of benefit from these interventions. This variability in treatment response poses a critical challenge in the management of anxiety disorders, often leading to prolonged suffering, increased healthcare costs, and reduced quality of life for those affected. The emerging paradigm of personalized medicine in mental health seeks to address these challenges by moving away from the one-size-fits-all approach to treatment. Instead, it emphasizes the importance of tailoring therapeutic strategies to the unique characteristics of each patient. This approach is particularly promising for anxiety disorders, where individual differences in biological, psychological, and environmental factors can significantly influence treatment outcomes (Lueken & Hahn, 2020). Machine learning and artificial intelligence (AI) technologies are at the forefront of this shift towards personalized medicine. These advanced technologies have the potential to revolutionize the way anxiety disorders are treated by enabling predictions on the individual patient level. AI thus can help in developing personalized treatment plans based on individual characteristics and preferences of the clients and can recommend tailored interventions based on the preferences, such as digital CBT, mindfulness exercises, or pharmacotherapy. Personalization enhances treatment adherence and effectiveness. In this context Ada Health is an AI-powered app that provides personalized health assessments and recommendations. It asks users about their symptoms, medical history, and preferences, and uses AI to generate individualized treatment plans for anxiety and other conditions.

Some other notable developments include the apps related to **Mindfulness and Relaxation**. These apps personalize meditation sessions and recommend specific exercises based on user data, e.g. Sanvello is a digital therapeutic app that uses AI to deliver CBT, mindfulness, and relaxation techniques. It offers personalized tools and resources to help users manage anxiety and stress, including mood tracking, guided meditations, and coping strategies.

Virtual Reality (VR) and Exposure Therapy: Some of the therapeutic techniques in management of anxiety disorders include exposure and response prevention or graded exposure, where the client is exposed to an unwanted situation or behaviour and is gradually moderated to achieve a desired level of response to the situation. The technique is effective in individuals with social anxiety, phobia, obsessive–compulsive disorder, and panic disorder. This exposure is done in two different ways, one imaginary or 'in-vitro'; and one in a real situation known as 'in-vivo'. In many circumstances, it is difficult to put clients in 'in vivo' exposure, and they might find it difficult engaging themselves in 'in- vitro' exposure. In these scenarios, virtual reality can be very handy, and AI can enhance VR therapy for anxiety disorders by creating immersive and interactive environments that simulate real-life situations. VR exposure therapy involves gradually exposing individuals to anxiety-provoking situations in a controlled environment. AI can personalize the experience by adjusting the intensity and duration of exposure based on the user's progress.

Social Skills Training: VR environments can also be used for social skill training as they can also simulate social interactions. Using VR-based therapy can help individuals with social anxiety practice and improve their social skills, e.g. Limbix VR offers VR-based exposure therapy for anxiety disorders. It uses AI to create realistic and customizable scenarios, such as public speaking or flying, allowing users to confront their fears in a safe and controlled setting.

Monitoring and Relapse Prevention

While anxiety disorders are pretty much amenable to psychotherapeutic management, relapse of symptoms are also common. It is a common observation that several patients upon certain improvement in their symptom levels, miss their regular follow-up, both for psychotherapeutic and pharmacotherapy, which is a big risk for relapse. Thus, therapeutic management will be incomplete without structured efforts for relapse prevention. One of the major factors for relapse not only in anxiety disorder rather most mental health conditions is inadequate monitoring in between follow ups and missed opportunities to identify early signs of relapse. Continuous monitoring is known to be tedious for caregivers and cause of burn out. AI can be helpful in this situation and provide continuous monitoring and support, and it can also minimize the need to visit the clinic physically by patient or family. The monitoring can be done through apps on wearable devices or even smartphones.

A major benefit of using smart apps is their 24/7 connectivity and for critical patients, it can send alerts to all concerned in real-time. The AI-powered wearable devices can track physiological markers, such as heart rate variability and sleep patterns, to monitor anxiety levels. These devices can alert users and their healthcare providers to early signs of relapse. Data can be analysed from smartphone apps to monitor changes in behaviour, mood, and activity levels too, providing real-time feedback and interventions to help users manage their anxiety. For example, Mindstrong Health uses AI to analyse data from smartphones, such as typing patterns and voice tone, to monitor mental health. It provides users with insights into their mental well-being and alerts them to potential changes in anxiety levels.

Digital Coaching and Support: As earlier mentioned, the aim of using AI in mental health care is not to replace human professionals but to aid them in enhancing their functionality, save time and provide access to more people. Individuals with anxiety disorder generally do have a fair level of insight, and many look for tutorial or self-help before consulting a professional. Preventive strategies like these can have a major effect on the progression of the illness, and thus AI has a big role to play here. AI can offer digital coaching and support to help individuals manage anxiety on a daily basis. AI chatbots can engage users in therapeutic conversations, offering support, guidance, and coping strategies. These chatbots are available 24/7, providing immediate assistance when needed. AI-powered virtual therapists can also offer personalized coaching and support through video or text-based interactions. They can help users develop and maintain healthy habits, such as regular exercise and relaxation techniques. For example, Wysa is an AI chatbot that provides digital coaching and support for anxiety and other mental health issues. It engages users in empathetic conversations and offers personalized tools and techniques to help manage anxiety, such as breathing exercises and cognitive restructuring. However, users must be aware of the limitations of these chatbots and virtual therapists and must not be used as an alternative to experienced mental health professionals.

AI Technologies for Predicting Treatment Response in Anxiety Disorders

As we discussed how AI is implicated in providing personalized treatment plans, such predictions allow clinicians to match patients with the interventions most likely to be effective for them, thereby maximizing the chances of a successful outcome. AI and machine learning algorithms work by analysing large and complex datasets that include a wide range of patient characteristics, such as genetic information, neuroimaging data, clinical histories, and even behavioural patterns captured through digital phenotyping. By identifying patterns and correlations within these datasets, AI systems can predict how a specific patient is likely to respond to various treatment options. This predictive capability represents a significant advancement over traditional approaches, which often rely on generalized treatment guidelines that may not account for individual differences. One of the most promising applications of AI in this context is the development of predictive models that can forecast a patient's response to specific psychotherapeutic or pharmacological treatments. For example, AI algorithms can analyse data from previous patients to identify which characteristics are associated with positive responses to cognitive-behavioural therapy (CBT) or particular antidepressant medications. This information can then be used to guide treatment decisions for new patients, helping clinicians select the most appropriate therapy from the outset.

AI technologies can continually refine these predictions as more data become available, making them increasingly accurate over time. This dynamic learning process allows for the ongoing improvement of treatment strategies, ensuring that they remain aligned with the latest scientific evidence and clinical practice. The integration of AI into the treatment of anxiety disorders also holds promise for addressing some of the current limitations in mental health care. For instance, AI-driven tools can assist in identifying patients who are at high risk of poor treatment outcomes or those who may benefit from more intensive or alternative interventions. This capability is particularly important for vulnerable patient groups, who are often underserved by traditional approaches to mental health care. The application of machine learning and AI technologies in the treatment of anxiety disorders represents a significant step forward in the field of personalized medicine. By enabling precise, data-driven predictions on the individual patient level, these technologies have the potential to improve treatment outcomes, reduce the trial-and-error process associated with finding effective therapies, and ultimately enhance the quality of care for individuals with anxiety disorders. As research and development in this area continue to advance, the future of anxiety disorder treatment looks increasingly personalized, effective, and responsive to the unique needs of each patient.

Major Innovations and Utility

Continued advancements in AI technology, such as deep learning and natural language processing, have enhanced the potentials and capabilities of AI tools for anxiety spectrum disorder treatment. These advancements will enable more accurate and personalized interventions. Currently, the algorithm models appear to focus on single disorders and are due to navigate the complications of overlapping symptoms and comorbid conditions, but the literature is promising. One of the major reasons why mental health conditions become chronic or less amenable to treatment is the delay in seeking treatment early, and anxiety disorders are no exception. But early identification on part of even clients might be difficult, as even they may be looking at their symptoms as part of their behavioural pattern. On top unless clients consult any professional, intervention is difficult, thus early identification is pretty difficult in such circumstances. However, AI can provide vital clues even before symptoms are florid for an individual, giving a valuable window for early intervention. At present much of the early identification, where clients are not formally engaged, is coming mostly from sentiment analysis of social media usage patterns, however the literature on this is sparse (Mansoor & Ansari, 2024), and data from wearable devices (Abd-Alrazaq et al., 2023). Even if these AI tools are in their preliminary stage, and desire refinement, there is no harm in taking precaution from alerts by these tools. What adds credibility to prediction models of AI, is its ability to analyse biological markers, such as genetic data, neuroimaging, and blood tests, to identify potential biomarkers associated with anxiety disorders. This can give early indications to users even before symptoms of the disorder become florid. AI algorithms can analyse text and speech data to identify linguistic patterns and markers associated with anxiety.

For example, increased use of negative language, pronouns like "I" or "me", and hesitation words may indicate anxiety.

Machine Learning Models: Machine learning models can be trained on large datasets to predict the likelihood of anxiety disorders based on various features, such as demographic information, medical history, and self-reported symptoms. Some of the most common and cited algorithms and categories include the Bayesian network, Artificial Neural Networks (ANN), Support Vector Machine (SVM), Decision trees, and Neuro-Fuzzy Systems (NFSs). Each of these methods enjoy different levels of accuracy levels of around 70–75%. Meta reviews suggest that ANNs managed to achieve the highest prediction score compared to the other methods used for the prediction of Generalized Anxiety Disorder. Further, hybrid methods and support vector machines (SVMs) were the most highly used methods especially for the prediction of Post-Traumatic Stress Disorder and Social Anxiety Disorder, respectively.

Transforming Conventional Anxiety Assessment with AI-Based Assessment and Monitoring

The Beck Anxiety Inventory (Beck et al., 1988) is one of the most widely used scales to assess anxiety symptoms. It is a 21 item self-report measure of anxiety with good psychometric properties. For the assessment, the patient is asked to rate the symptoms which have been bothering him during the past month as per its severity. However, the scale is often criticized for its limitation of having difficulty in discriminating between anxiety and depression in a primary care population, as the symptoms may be present in milder forms of depression too. In this scenario, AI-augmented BAI rating can give a more reliable impression of the anxiety symptoms and help discriminate it from depressive illness. The following 21 symptoms of anxiety disorders, assessed by the BAI scale, can be better evaluated, tracked, and monitored using AI-based tools (Table 5.1). Such tools can utilize natural language processing (NLP), wearable devices, and other technologies for real-time assessment. The benefit of the AI-augmented assessment would be, it can give a timeline of each of the specific symptoms through quantifiable data, and does not rely on patients' memory, nullifying scope of biased rating or error due to lack of understanding by the patient.

While this augmentation of AI for reliable quantification of anxiety symptoms is one step; in future, a more diverse assessment tool can be made using AI, incorporating socio-cultural influencers and determinants specific to each patient.

Table 5.1 AI-based assessment of anxiety symptoms (based on BAI items)

Symptoms	AI-based assessment method
Numbness or tingling	Monitored using wearable sensors that detect changes in skin conductivity or peripheral nerve signals
Feeling hot	Detected via temperature sensors in wearable devices or self-reported through chatbot queries
Wobbliness in legs	Identified through gait analysis using motion-sensing wearables or phone accelerometers
Unable to relax	Assessed using NLP in chatbot interactions to identify signs of restlessness or tension in user responses
Fear of worst happening	Evaluated using conversational AI to detect catastrophic thought patterns in user dialogues
Dizzy or lightheaded	Tracked via wearable devices that monitor blood pressure and balance or reported via chatbot queries
Heart pounding / racing	Measured using heart rate variability (HRV) data from fitness trackers or smartwatches
Unsteady	Identified through posture analysis using accelerometers in wearables or mobile apps
Terrified or afraid	Detected using emotional sentiment analysis from user responses in conversational AI
Nervous	Analysed through voice emotion analysis or NLP-based interpretation of anxiety-related language
Feeling of choking	Monitored using respiration rate sensors embedded in wearable devices
Hands trembling	Tracked using motion sensors in wearables or user-reported in chatbot interactions
Shaky/unsteady	Measured via accelerometers to detect hand or body tremors
Fear of losing control	Evaluated using chatbot-based conversational prompts to assess cognitive distortions or irrational fears
Difficulty in breathing	Monitored using respiratory sensors or self-reports during chatbot assessments
Fear of dying	Identified through sentiment analysis of self-reported concerns or thought patterns via AI chatbots
Scared	Assessed using emotion recognition from text or voice inputs
Indigestion	Tracked using self-reports or AI-enabled health-tracking apps linked to dietary and digestive patterns
Faint / lightheaded	Detected through wearable monitoring of blood pressure or user-reported in conversations
Face flushed	Identified via wearable cameras or thermographic sensors monitoring facial temperature changes
Hot / cold sweats	Monitored using skin conductivity sensors (electrodermal activity) or user reports in AI chatbots

The Road Ahead

AI need not be looked upon as the independent future in mental health and need to be integrated with conventional evidence-based therapies only. Even though it will take some time, AI tools are likely to be integrated and in fact need to be integrated with traditional therapy, like psychoeducation, CBT enhancing the overall treatment experience. This will assist therapists by providing real-time insights and recommendations based on patient data, complementing in-person sessions. While initial sessions can be in clinic set up, follow-up can be assisted by AI on need basis with due assistance in monitoring, and helping in preventing relapse.

Multimodal Approaches: Future AI interventions will likely adopt multimodal approaches, combining various data sources, such as text, speech, and physiological data, which will help symptoms tracking, associated triggers and causal factors, to provide a comprehensive understanding of anxiety disorders. This will enable more accurate diagnosis and personalized treatment. AI has significant potential regarding early identification by using large data and using it in community awareness too.

Collaborative Efforts: The development and deployment of AI tools for anxiety spectrum disorder treatment will require collaborative efforts among researchers, clinicians, developers, and policymakers. Multidisciplinary approaches will ensure that AI interventions are evidence-based, ethical, and aligned with user needs.

Conclusion

AI has huge potential to transform the diagnosis, treatment, and management of anxiety spectrum disorders. By leveraging AI technology, mental health care can become more accessible, cost-effective, and personalized. With refinement and advancement AI models are gradually becoming more efficient in providing information for early identification, diagnosis as well as management. However, the deployment of AI in this field must be guided by ethical considerations and evidence-based practices to ensure safety, effectiveness, and user satisfaction. As technology continues to advance, AI will play an increasingly important role in enhancing mental health care and improving outcomes for individuals with anxiety spectrum disorders.

References

Abd-Alrazaq, A., AlSaad, R., Harfouche, M., Aziz, S., Ahmed, A., Damseh, R., & Sheikh, J. (2023). Wearable artificial intelligence for detecting anxiety: Systematic review and meta-analysis. *Journal of Medical Internet Research, 25*, Article e48754. https://doi.org/10.2196/48754

Beck, A. T., Epstein, N., Brown, G., & Steer, R. A. (1988). An inventory for measuring clinical anxiety: Psychometric properties. *Journal of Consulting and Clinical Psychology, 56*, 893–897.

Brown, K. (2021, June 1). Something bothering you? Tell it to Woebot. *The New York Times*. Retrieved November 15, 2024, from https://www.nytimes.com/2021/06/01/health/artificial-intelligence-therapy-woebot.html.

Carter, R. M., Wittchen, H. U., Pfister, H., & Kessler, R. C. (2001). One-year prevalence of subthreshold and threshold DSM-IV generalized anxiety disorder in a nationally representative sample. *Depression and Anxiety, 13*(2), 78–88. https://doi.org/10.1002/da.1020

Chang, X., Gong, Q., Li, C., Yue, W., Yu, X., Yao, S., & Feng, J. (2021). Psychiatric disorders in China: Strengths and challenges of contemporary research and clinical services. *Psychological Medicine, 51*(12), 1978–1991. https://doi.org/10.1017/S0033291721002816

Eltahawy, L., Essig, T., Myszkowski, N., & Trub, L. (2024). Can robots do therapy? Examining the efficacy of a CBT bot in comparison with other behavioral intervention technologies in alleviating mental health symptoms. *Computers in Human Behavior: Artificial Humans, 2*(1), 1–14. https://doi.org/10.1016/j.chbah.2023.100035

Lueken, U., & Hahn, T. (2020). Personalized mental health: Artificial intelligence technologies for treatment response prediction in anxiety disorders. In B. T. Baun (Ed.), *Personalized Psychiatry* (pp. 201–213). Academic Press.

Maier, W., Buller, R., Philipp, M., & Heuser, I. (1988). The Hamilton anxiety scale: Reliability, validity and sensitivity to change in anxiety and depressive disorders. *Journal of Affective Disorders, 14*(1), 61–68. https://doi.org/10.1016/0165-0327(88)90072-9

Mansoor, M. A., & Ansari, K. H. (2024). Early detection of mental health crises through artificial-intelligence-powered social media analysis: A prospective observational study. *Journal of Personalized Medicine, 14*, 958. https://doi.org/10.3390/jpm14090958

Martin, D. C. (1990). The mental status examination. In H. K. Walker, W. D. Hall, & J. W. Hurst (Eds.), *Clinical methods: The history, physical, and laboratory examinations* (3rd ed., Chapter 207). Butterworths. https://www.ncbi.nlm.nih.gov/books/NBK320/.

Muntingh, A. D., van der Feltz-Cornelis, C. M., van Marwijk, H. W., Spinhoven, P., Penninx, B. W., & van Balkom, A. J. (2011). Is the Beck Anxiety Inventory a good tool to assess the severity of anxiety? A primary care study in the Netherlands Study of Depression and Anxiety (NESDA). *BMC Family Practice, 12*, 66. https://doi.org/10.1186/1471-2296-12-66

Wittchen, H. U., Zhao, S., Kessler, R. C., & Eaton, W. W. (1994). DSM-III-R generalized anxiety disorder in the National Comorbidity Survey. *Archives of General Psychiatry, 51*(5), 355–364. https://doi.org/10.1001/archpsyc.1994.03950050015002

Chapter 6
AI in Mood Disorders and Suicide Risk

Abstract Mood disorders, including depression and bipolar disorder, are among the most common and debilitating mental health conditions. These disorders not only impair the quality of life of suffering individuals, but also are major risk of suicide, which is a leading cause of death worldwide. Traditional methods of diagnosing and treating mood disorders though appear to be effective; they often face limitations in terms of accessibility, cost and personalization. On other hand suicide prevention remains a very delicate issue. Artificial Intelligence (AI) has emerged as a promising tool to address these challenges, offering innovative solutions for early detection, treatment, and ongoing management of mood disorders and suicide risk. This chapter explores the role of AI in addressing mood disorders and suicide prevention, highlighting various applications, benefits, limitations, and future directions in this field.

Keywords Mood disorders · Depression · Suicide risk · Mood tracker

Understanding Mood Disorders and Suicide

Mood disorders encompass a range of mental health conditions characterized by significant disturbances in a person's mood. The major categories of mood disorders include:

- Major Depressive Disorder (MDD): It is characterized by persistent feelings of sadness, loss of interest or pleasure in activities, and various cognitive and physical symptoms.
- Bipolar Disorder: It involves episodes of mania or hypomania (elevated mood and energy) alternating with episodes of depression.
- Persistent Depressive Disorder (Dysthymia): A chronic form of depression in lesser severity with symptoms lasting for at least two years.
- Cyclothymic Disorder: A milder form of bipolar disorder with less severe mood swings.

S. Halder et al., *Navigating AI in Mental Health Care*,
https://doi.org/10.1007/978-981-96-9744-1_6

For many, mood disorders are synonymous to depression only; however, clinical disturbances in mood can happen in several ways including manic manifestation in which the individual has elated mood, inflated self-esteem, coupled with high energy levels, disturbed sleep pattern, increased talk, etc. Severe forms of both mania and depression can be accompanied with features of psychosis. The categories listed above are not exhaustive as per both the DSM and the ICD.

Suicide on other hand is defined as death caused by self-directed injurious behaviour with intent to die as a result of the behaviour. People generally associate suicide as an abrupt outcome as an individual's reaction to certain stress, but this may not be true. It is true that presence of mental illness increases the risk of suicide in an individual manifold, and individuals with major depressive disorder are at a higher risk of suicidality, compared to others.

Prevalence

Mood disorders are considered as major mental illnesses and affect millions of individuals globally, leading to substantial personal, social, and economic burdens. They impair daily functioning, relationships, and productivity, and are associated with high rates of comorbidity with other mental and physical health conditions. An estimated 3.8% of the population experience depression, including 5% of adults (4% among men and 6% among women), and 5.7% of adults older than 60 years. This corresponds to approximately 280 million people in the world having depression (IHME, 2021). What is worrisome is the fact that the prevalence of major depressive episodes was higher among adult females (10.3%) compared to males (6.2%). Further, the prevalence of adults with a major depressive episode was highest among individuals aged 18–25 (18.6%). While this data is relevant to the United States for the year 2021, the pattern of data would be more or less similar with minor variations in other countries.

In contrast, figures for suicide are much higher when compared to depressive disorders. As per the World Health Organization (WHO) more than 700 000 people die globally by suicide every year, which is about one person every 40 s. In the year 2019, 77% of suicides occurred in low- and middle-income countries, accounting for 1.3% of all deaths worldwide making it the 17th leading cause of death. The fact that numbers of suicide is much higher than numbers of people with depressive illnesses is clear indication of the heterogeneous causes behind suicide. However, depressive illness remains a major risk, as the US National Comorbidity Survey found the risk of suicide attempts five-fold higher in patients with major depressive disorder than in the general population (Nock et al., 2010). Patients with a major depressive episode have increased risk of completed suicide after suicidal attempts (Suominen et al, 2009).

Conventional Diagnostic and Treatment Approaches: Management of mood disorders frequently include prescription drugs, medical advice, and continuing specialized supervision. A major component includes individual and supportive psychotherapy, which helps suffering individuals to cope with their stressors, identify early signs of relapse, and relapse prevention, as well as counter suicidal thoughts.

Identifying Depression and Its Determinants upon Initiating Treatment

1. **Primary care providers** often serve as the first point of contact for individuals experiencing depression, playing a critical role in initiating appropriate therapeutic strategies. These physicians are typically the first to recognize depressive symptoms, whether by diagnosing and beginning treatment or by referring patients to mental health specialists according to established guidelines. Accurate diagnosis and treatment are paramount for ensuring continuity of care, and the longstanding relationship between family physicians and their patients can significantly enhance therapeutic outcomes through mutual trust and easier access to care. This relationship allows primary care providers to follow clinical guidelines more effectively, offering standardized and high-quality care while reducing inconsistencies in treatment outcomes.
2. The treatment approaches taken by primary care providers are primarily influenced by **clinical recommendations and guidelines** of relevant medical bodies, which are more or less uniform as per evidence base of treatment approaches. These guidelines, which are evidence-based, provide a structured approach to diagnosing and managing major depressive disorder (MDD). They often recommend a stepped-care approach, beginning with minimally invasive interventions such as psychoeducation and close monitoring for milder cases. For more severe cases, the guidelines suggest escalating to psychological therapies and pharmacological interventions. By adhering to these guidelines, primary care providers can deliver consistent and effective care, mitigating the variability often observed in treatment outcomes.
3. **Various patient characteristics**, including the severity of depression, comorbid medical conditions, previous treatment history, and personal preferences, significantly influence the therapeutic decisions made by primary care providers. For instance, patients exhibiting severe depression or those who are unresponsive to initial treatments may require more aggressive therapeutic interventions, such as a combination of antidepressants and psychotherapy. Additionally, individual preferences can guide primary care providers in selecting specific treatment modalities, emphasizing the importance of patient-centred care in managing depression.
4. Extensive research supports the efficacy of both psychotherapy and antidepressant medications in treating depression. Treatment guidelines recommend the continuous use of antidepressants for several months to achieve and maintain

remission. However, despite these recommendations, only about half of individuals with depression receive adequate treatment. This gap in treatment provision can be attributed to several factors, including the underdiagnosis of depression in primary care settings, the limited availability of outpatient psychotherapists, and the inadequate adherence of some therapists to evidence-based interventions. Consequently, many patients with mild to moderate depressive symptoms are often prescribed antidepressant medications alone, a practice that deviates from the recommended guidelines of combined approach of psychotherapy and pharmacotherapy which always has a better outcome.

5. **The accuracy of depression diagnoses** made by primary care physicians has been a subject of concern. The positive predictive value of these diagnoses is approximately 42%, indicating that 58% of identified cases may be false positives (Mitchell et al., 2011). This statistic suggests that a significant proportion of antidepressant prescriptions written by primary care physicians are for patients with mild depression, including those with subthreshold symptoms. In fact, the majority (60–85%) of these prescriptions are for treating depression in adults, with only a minority prescribed for other conditions. However, this gap may not always be attributed to the consultant, but factors like unavailability of reliable information, inadequate reporting on part of client may also play a role in this. In Europe and the United States, an estimated 5–16% of adults are prescribed antidepressants annually. Thus, AI has a potential role in improving these figures.
6. **The competence and education of primary care practitioners** play a significant role in their clinical decision-making processes. More experienced physicians tend to be more confident in diagnosing depression and initiating treatment, whereas less experienced providers may more frequently refer patients to specialists. Several factors can negatively impact adherence to depression management guidelines, including patient-related factors, professional constraints, and systemic issues within healthcare organizations. For instance, patients may deny experiencing symptoms of depression and instead seek help for physical complaints, which can complicate the diagnostic process. Additionally, a psychiatric diagnosis does not always guarantee that either the patient or the physician will view treatment as necessary.
7. Primary care physicians may face challenges in adhering to guidelines due to difficulties in distinguishing between normal distress and actual anxiety or depressive disorders. Moreover, some physicians may struggle to discuss sensitive aspects of a depression diagnosis with their patients. Organizational factors, such as inadequate collaboration between primary care providers and mental health specialists, long waiting lists for specialized mental health services, and insufficient financial incentives, can also hinder compliance with treatment guidelines. AI can facilitate better and real-time coordination between different centres for better referral systems for effective patient management.
8. While **patient diversity** undeniably contributes to variability in treatment outcomes, emerging evidence highlights the significant impact of differences in physicians' decision-making processes. For example, research has shown

considerable variation in physicians' beliefs about the most appropriate treatment course. Survey data indicate that most physicians exhibit a preference for a particular drug, and on average, their preferred medication accounts for an average of 66% of their overall prescriptions. AI can assist clinicians in choosing among the best options available as well as suitable to the client.

9. **The perspectives and beliefs of primary care** physicians can greatly influence patients' willingness to disclose their issues, thereby affecting the initial identification of depressive symptoms, subsequent therapeutic decisions, and the adoption of new approaches in clinical practice. Clinicians' attitudes towards mental illness may reflect common societal stereotypes and misconceptions, shaped by their personal experiences and professional training. A lack of specificity in depression screening among primary care physicians can lead to misdiagnosis, where individuals without depression are incorrectly identified as having the disorder. This issue is particularly prevalent in the misdiagnosis of depression among female, elderly, and racial minority patients. Such overdiagnoses can impose an unnecessary treatment burden on the healthcare system, leading to wasted resources and the inappropriate use of health services.
10. **Overdiagnosis of depression** can also result in healthy individuals being erroneously diagnosed and treated, leading to potential iatrogenic effects from unnecessary treatments. This issue underscores the importance of addressing and countering power imbalances in the clinical relationship. Research has extensively documented implicit biases related to race, ethnicity, sociodemographic factors, and gender among primary care physicians. For instance, studies have found that female patients, unemployed individuals, those with limited education, and those with lower incomes are more likely to be diagnosed with mental health problems. Conversely, patients with higher socioeconomic status are more likely to engage in meaningful conversations with their physicians, potentially leading to more accurate diagnoses and appropriate treatments.
11. Moreover, evidence suggests that **gender disparities** exist in how physicians' approach common somatic symptoms. Men who present with such symptoms are more likely to undergo physical examinations, diagnostic imaging, and specialist referrals compared to women with similar complaints. These findings highlight the need for greater awareness of and strategies to mitigate biases in clinical practice to ensure equitable treatment for all patients.

In this context, artificial intelligence (AI) tools, such as ChatGPT, offer several advantages over traditional primary care and even mental health professionals in detecting depression (Levkovich et al., 2023). ChatGPT can provide objective, data-driven insights that complement conventional diagnostic methods. It has the ability to analyse large datasets quickly, facilitating early detection and intervention. Additionally, ChatGPT offers confidentiality and anonymity, which may encourage patients to seek help without fear of stigma or professional repercussions. This capability could be particularly valuable in addressing the underdiagnosis and misdiagnosis of depression in primary care settings, ultimately improving treatment outcomes for a diverse patient population.

Issues with Diagnosing Mood Disorders

It's a fact that all of us do get affected by setbacks in life and have experienced low moods on and off in our lives. However, most people recover from them gradually and are back to their usual routine soon. But low mood due to clinical depression may not be secondary to any setback in life and may look like usual mood fluctuations when in early stages. They are difficult to be gauged, thus even if family members notice one of their members withdrawn for a while, they might console or comfort him but are less likely to think of it as depression at first instance. Further, unless severe, symptoms of depression are less likely to be accompanied with physical symptoms, which does not warrant immediate medical attention to family members or the individual himself, causing delay in first consultation for patients with depressive illness. Diagnosis of mood disorders typically depends on clinical judgement of the professional, and does not include any validation of biomarkers, as there are none established as of now. The overlapping of symptoms and presence of comorbid conditions, which are pretty common, make diagnostic decisions a bit difficult in absence of reliable clinical history.

Early Detection and Diagnosis of Mood Disorders with Help of AI

AI has the potential to improve depression prognosis and early diagnosis. By analysing vast datasets—including genetic information, patient medical records, and social media activity—AI algorithms can identify individuals at risk of depression and differentiate them from the general population (Graham et al., 2019). This capability allows for timely interventions and preventive measures. AI can be instrumental in refining treatment strategies for depression, offering a more personalized and effective approach to mental health care (Fig. 6.1). Psychological depression is being explored as a potential target for advanced artificial intelligence (AI) interventions. AI has demonstrated considerable potential in revolutionizing the diagnosis, monitoring, and treatment of depression through its ability to analyse large volumes of data and identify patterns indicative of mental health conditions. By employing sophisticated algorithms and machine learning techniques, AI can enhance the effectiveness of treatment programmes by delivering personalized interventions.

Use of screening tools for assessment of mood is common like other mental health conditions. These tools require a certain level of discretion and selection on part of the therapist when done in face-to-face sessions; however, these tools may be corroborated with mood trackers so that a self-rating can be obtained and indicate presence and severity of manic or depressive symptoms. It will remain challenging though, how the information or how much of this information will be shared with the user in a non-threatening way and initiate corrective measures.

While Natural Language Processing (NLP) and Machine Learning remain the tested tools for assisting in the diagnosis as well as monitoring patients with mood disorders, analysing behavioural patterns can drop a big hint in the purpose. AI, particularly NLP, can analyse language patterns in text and speech to detect symptoms of mood disorders. By examining linguistic markers such as word choice, sentence structure, and speech rhythm, AI can identify signs of depression or mania. AI tools can analyse social media posts, emails, and journal entries to detect language patterns indicative of mood disorders. For instance, excessive use of negative words, pronouns like "I" or "me", and expressions of "hopelessness" or "worthlessness" can signal depression. On the other hand, machine learning algorithms models can integrate data from multiple sources, including electronic health records, wearable devices, and self-report surveys to predict the onset of mood disorders. Predictive Analytics Platforms like Mindstrong Health utilize machine learning to analyse data from smartphones and wearables, such as typing patterns, voice tone, and physical activity, to predict mood disorder episodes and provide early intervention.

Physiological and Behavioural Monitoring is an important aspect in mood disorders: AI can analyse physiological and behavioural data to detect early signs of mood disorders. Wearable devices and smartphones can track metrics such as heart rate variability, sleep patterns, and physical activity levels, which are often disrupted in mood disorders. Any change in the usual parameters may be used to alert users to take preventive steps, and the data may be shared later with professionals for tracking. Smart wearable devices like Fitbit and Apple Watch can collect continuous physiological data, which AI algorithms can analyse to detect deviations from baseline that may indicate mood disturbances.

Case Example of a Lady with Bipolar Affective Disorder

We take an example of a 35-year-old housewife, diagnosed with Bipolar Affective Disorder, presented with multiple episodes of both mania and depression for more than 8 years. Though she is under psychiatric treatment, compliance to medication as well as psychotherapy sessions had been irregular. She tends to miss follow-ups for medication as well as psychotherapy sessions once symptoms improve and are maintained for a while upon nearing premorbid levels. She would further consult again when symptoms resurface in an episodic manner, and with increased severity. Though hailing from a financially well-off family, family members and direct caregivers appeared having divided opinion and understanding of the patient's illness and the need of both pharmacological and psychological intervention. Psychoeducation was provided to the patient as well as caregivers, detailing the episodic nature of illness, symptom manifestation, course and progression. They were also detailed about the relapsing nature of the illness and advised on its early identification. Despite these, the treatment compliance was not satisfactory and there was relapse.

Cases like this are common in psychiatric setups. While psychoeducation is an effective tool to enhance insight of patients and caregivers having direct impact on treatment compliance and outcome, in certain cases some extra inputs like mood trackers are desired. One of the easy but reliable desired self-help techniques is use of mood trackers. Mood trackers have been used even before the advent of AI, but a well-structured psychoeducation, adjunct with AI-assisted mood tracker can make significant impact by reducing relapse rates.

AI-Assisted Mood Tracking

Mood tracking or mood monitoring is a crucial self-help method for patients with mood disorders, in which they keep a track of their mood states at regular intervals, also noting the antecedent circumstances, any observable triggers. The process has been beneficial for patients in understanding the pattern of their mood variations and its likely triggers, which helped in the therapy process. However, with advancements in AI, these mood trackers have moved from paper–pencil to wearable devices as well as smartphones, which provide a better accounting of the mood tracking. Even though the issue of subjective bias remains to a certain extent, these devices can also measure physiological arousal or other physiological responses to corroborate with the reported mood state, providing a more accurate account. There are already mood tracker apps available to users, including ‘Breath’, ‘Wysa’, and ‘Kintsugi. Some of these are also capable of mood tracking by reading users’ facial micro-expressions throughout the day and generating beautiful infographics to help them visualize their moods over time. Augmentation of AI for enhanced and effective mood tracking and early detection.

Effectiveness of an AI-Enhanced Clinical Decision Support System in Depression Treatment

The idea of introducing AI in clinical decision-making is not to influence the clinical judgement of clinicians, rather to provide a neutral feedback and analysis of available data, which may go unnoticed by the clinician and help him/her in effective decision-making. The integration of Artificial Intelligence (AI) into health care has opened new avenues for improving the diagnosis and treatment of mental health disorders, particularly depression. One significant advancement is the development of AI-enhanced Clinical Decision Support Systems (CDSS), which offer promising tools for enhancing the effectiveness and efficiency of depression treatment (Benrimoh et al., 2018). These systems leverage AI algorithms to analyse complex datasets, providing clinicians with evidence-based recommendations that can optimize patient outcomes. AI-enhanced CDSS for depression treatment operates by processing vast amounts of patient data, including medical history, genetic

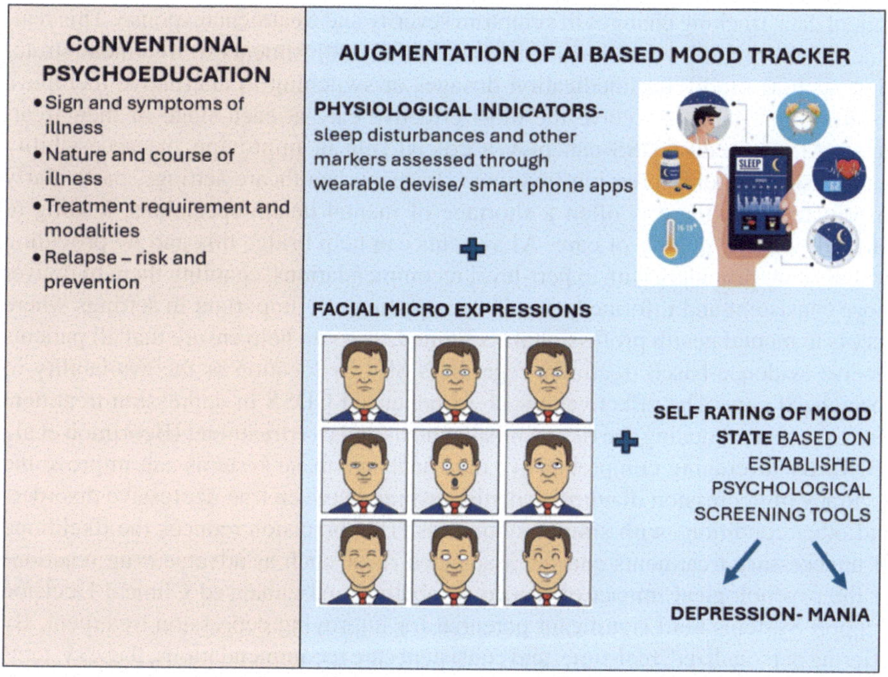

Fig. 6.1 Augmentation of AI for enhanced and effective mood tracking and early detection. Image credit: freepik.com

information, symptomatology, and even behavioural patterns gathered from electronic health records (EHRs). By doing so, these systems can identify patterns and correlations that may not be immediately apparent to human clinicians. This capability is particularly valuable in the context of depression, a multifaceted disorder influenced by a combination of biological, psychological, and social factors. One of the key benefits of AI-powered CDSS is its ability to personalize treatment plans (Cerrato & Halamka, 2020). Traditional approaches to depression treatment often rely on standardized protocols, which may not account for the unique characteristics of each patient. In contrast, AI-enhanced systems can tailor treatment recommendations based on individual patient profiles. For example, the system might suggest specific antidepressants or psychotherapy approaches that are more likely to be effective for a particular patient, based on their unique clinical presentation and history. This personalized approach can reduce the trial-and-error period often associated with finding the right treatment, thereby improving patient outcomes and reducing the overall burden of the disorder.

Another significant advantage of AI-enhanced CDSS is its capacity for real-time monitoring and adjustment of treatment plans. Depression is a dynamic condition, with symptoms that can fluctuate over time. AI systems can continuously analyse patient data, tracking changes in symptom severity and treatment response. This real-time monitoring allows clinicians to make timely adjustments to treatment strategies, such as modifying medication dosages or switching to alternative therapies, ensuring that patients receive the most effective care at each stage of their treatment. AI-enhanced CDSS can play a crucial role in improving the accessibility and consistency of depression treatment. In many healthcare settings, particularly in primary care, there is often a shortage of mental health specialists, leading to variability in the quality of care. AI systems can help bridge this gap by providing primary care providers with expert-level recommendations, enabling them to deliver more consistent and informed care. This is particularly important in settings where access to mental health professionals is limited, as it can help ensure that all patients receive evidence-based treatment regardless of their location or the availability of specialized care. The effectiveness of AI-enhanced CDSS in depression treatment also extends to reducing the risk of misdiagnosis and overtreatment (Benrimoh et al., 2018). By leveraging comprehensive data analysis, these systems can improve the accuracy of depression diagnoses, distinguishing between true depressive disorders and other conditions with similar symptoms. This precision reduces the likelihood of unnecessary treatments and the associated risks, such as adverse drug reactions or the psychological impact of incorrect labelling. AI-enhanced Clinical Decision Support Systems hold significant potential for improving depression treatment. By offering personalized, real-time, and consistent care recommendations, these systems can enhance patient outcomes, streamline treatment processes, and expand access to high-quality mental health care. As the technology continues to evolve, the role of AI in mental health care is likely to become increasingly prominent, paving the way for more effective and efficient treatment strategies for depression and other mental health disorders.

AI in the Treatment of Mood Disorders

The two major ways by which AI can aid in effective treatment for mood disorders are the scope of personalized treatment, and early identification and relapse prevention.

Personalized Treatment Plans: AI can help develop personalized treatment plans tailored to an individual's specific needs and preferences. By analysing patient data, AI can recommend the most effective treatment modalities, such as medication, psychotherapy, or lifestyle interventions. Integration of AI in treatment of mood disorders has opened new opportunities, as the method is very handy in tracking fluctuation in mood symptoms and mental state, providing a valuable window for timely intervention. For example, AI-driven platforms like Quartet Health analyse patient data to provide personalized treatment recommendations, integrating clinical assessments, patient history, and current symptoms to tailor interventions for mood disorders. These tools can provide cognitive-behavioural therapy (CBT), mindfulness exercises, and other therapeutic techniques. AI-Powered Therapy Apps like Woebot and Wysa deliver CBT and other therapeutic interventions. These apps engage users in therapeutic conversations, offering real-time support, feedback, and coping strategies to manage mood disorders.

Virtual Reality (VR) Therapy: While VR-based therapy have universal application, and predominantly used for anxiety spectrum disorder, they can provide immersive and interactive experiences for individuals with mood disorders also. VR environments can simulate real-life situations, helping users practice coping strategies and improve mood regulation. They can also be used for social skills practice in a controlled virtual environment.

Monitoring and Relapse Prevention: One of the major implications of AI for mood disorders would be in symptom monitoring and preventing relapse in between follow-up periods. Owing to the nature of mood disorders, particularly bipolar affective disorders are very likely to recur. This may happen, even when patients are fully compliant to treatment, and in major probability happen due to biogenetic propensity of the individual. Thus, identifying early symptoms of relapse, coupled with established biomarkers if any can indicate relapse even before symptoms reappear in full severity. We already discussed the use of mood tracker in the previous section that is valuable for preventing relapse. Platforms like Ginger.io use AI to monitor mental health continuously, analysing data from various sources to detect early signs of relapse and provide timely interventions.

AI in Suicide Prevention

Suicide may be secondary to certain mood disorders but also happen due to other independent causes. Committing suicide may look like a solitary incident, however it has different components as suicidality comprises suicidal ideation, suicide plan, suicide attempt, and completed suicide. Ideation refers to thoughts or wishes about ending one's life, plan refers to making plans for suicide, and attempt refers to acts to end one's life (Posner et al, 2007). Suicide attempt may happen without suicide plan, and all suicide ideations may not turn into suicide attempt. Since there is no cure of completed suicide, the only way out is preventing suicide, where understanding suicide behaviour in context of individual patient is important. Research in the domain suggest that risk factors for suicide vary widely and may include age group, sex, demographic profile, psychosocial support, presence of psychiatric morbidity or even physical illness (Halder & Mahato, 2016; Hua et al, 2024; Kerkhof & Arensman, 2000; Park et al, 2020). Even though there are numerous suicide helplines, there is still some gap as suicides continue to occur. Some of these deaths may be attributed to failure to reach the victim on time during his crisis, and failure to identify the crisis on time. AI can help in starting from identification of behaviour using large data to chatbot facilities for crisis management.

Continuous monitoring of individuals at risk of suicide is crucial for preventing repeat attempts. One of the factors why conventional suicide prevention fails is individuals in concern often do not confide in time or care givers fail to recognize warning signs. To some extent AI can add up to this monitoring for suicide risk by analysing data from wearable devices and smartphones to detect changes in behaviour or mood that may indicate increased suicide risk.

There is credible literature on use of AI been used for prediction of suicidal behaviour. Much of this literature bank on data from sentiment analysis of social media content and post of users (Aldhyani et al., 2022; Ramírez et al., 2020; Yeskuatov et al, 2022; Tadesse et al, 2020) but is not exhaustive and also include electronic health records from wearable devices.

Predictive models can identify individuals at high risk of suicide and trigger early intervention. Further tools like the Columbia-Suicide Severity Rating Scale (C-SSRS) can be augmented with AI to analyse patient responses and identify high-risk individuals.

Crisis Intervention and Support: One of the major benefits of using AI has been its use as programmable chatbots for suicide prevention. We discussed about the disturbing figures regarding suicide in previous section. Considering its public impact, there are numerous helplines which offer real-time support to individuals having suicidal thoughts and are actually doing a great work. But many such individuals who are at verge of engaging suicide attempt, may not give thought to discuss anything with other person. The reason could be anything including lack of trust in people, extreme sense of hopelessness, or considering their issues too private to discuss with an unknown person. If not all, some portion of these individuals might feel comfortable to share their thoughts of distress before engaging into suicide attempt. AI chatbots and virtual therapists in these conditions can provide immediate support and intervention for individuals experiencing suicidal thoughts. These tools can offer crisis counselling, advise strategies deterring suicidal behaviour and connections to emergency services. With refinement these chatbots may have the capacity to respond through text as well as speech. It is expected that the individual using these chatbots must be using it for a significant period of time, thus the bot does not necessarily wait for the user to share his suicidal thoughts but can analyse user data to identify risk and take pre-emptive measures.

Crisis Chat Bots like Crisis Text Line use AI to engage users in crisis situations, providing empathetic support and connecting them to human counsellors when needed. These chatbots can offer real-time assistance and help de-escalate suicidal crises.

Case Study

Miss M is a 21-year-old female. She is a college student and presented with complaints of low mood, reduced sleep and appetite, being withdrawn, crying spells, and repeated thoughts of committing suicide. The symptoms have been there for the past one and half year, with phases when she is relatively better. She attempted committing suicide twice in between and has been on medications.

Sample Talk:

Therapist: So, M, please tell me more. How did it start?

M: I joined this college two years back and have been staying in the students' accommodation. Shifted to this city and had difficulties adjusting with studies and friends…I feel very lonely, and left out….

Therapist: Do you have anyone or any friend to share your problems?

M: I don't have many friends, but J was really nice to me. I liked him but for him I was just a friend.

Therapist: Ok. Did you ever express your feelings towards Jacob?

M: I tried, but it seems he didn't take it seriously and asked me to focus on studies…

Therapist: did you try?

M: I tried...but can't...negative thoughts coming to my mind...to the extent that I am not good at studies. Can't make friends…I'm a failure…and I started thinking of killing myself...

Therapist: did it come before also, before joining college?

M: yes…in school, before board exams…but then I didn't attempt…this time it's too strong and I actually tried to kill myself…

Therapist: anyone came to know about it…

M: After they found the cut mark in my hand and blood coming out…

Therapist: Do you really want to kill yourself…

M: I regret, but if the situation does not improve, I don't know what I will do to cope with it…

….and conversation continues….

Clients like Miss M are frequent in outpatient clinics. Even though a significant number of them report improvement after therapy sessions, a certain number of them maintain a stable course. One of the probable factors could be failure to elicit the risk factors or trigger in these clients. This could be due to inadequate rapport development between the client and the therapist, or maybe the client himself does not deem certain situations as risk factors. Thus, the identification of risk factors is very important for patients with suicidal behaviour.

If we look at the trend, data analysis of content on social media is primarily used by AI programmes for detection of suicide risk in users, and there is a growing body of encouraging literature on it (Castillo et al. 2020; Cheng et al, 2017; Lekkas & Jacobson, 2023). Even if the literature is showing an increasing efficacy of AI capability in predicting suicide behaviour, social media content relatively has less face value compared to real clinical data. Thus, it could be desired that AI data from predictive analysis is added up with data from patients who have engaged in suicide behaviour in actual. These data can be gathered following ethical clearance and informed consent from clinics and hospitals and can add credible value to existing data pools.

Following is sample verbatim from actual clients with suicidal behaviour or ideation or attempt (Halder & Mahato, Unpublished).

"I am useless"; "I feel ignored by all"; "I am not worth"; "No one understands me"; "What if I am not here. Nothing changes"; "No point living"; "Can't bear the pain"; "Don't know how I will manage this"; "I just want to die"; " What's the point of living"; "Seems death is the solution"; "Others are suffering because of me"

When put into an algorithm, they are capable of highlighting specific words which are frequently expressed by individuals with suicide behaviour (Fig. 6.2).

Adding this kind of real data with predictive data could be a time-taking task as these predictive models require large data, there is a possibility of adding standard screening measures to smartphone apps, which when rated can give credible corroboration with user's suicidal ideations. These in turn may add new data for predictive analysis. One issue however remains how the technology can be used for real-time prevention, as even individuals who are identified at risk may perceive this as breach of their data privacy.

Benefits of AI in Mood Disorders and Suicide Prevention

Even though there are numerous helplines and mental health clinics, AI-assisted interventions can add value to existing service patterns.

Enhanced Accessibility: AI-powered tools can increase access to mental health care for individuals who face barriers to traditional therapy, such as geographical location, cost, or stigma. Digital therapeutics and AI chatbots can provide support to individuals who may not have access to in-person services.

Timely Interventions: AI can provide timely interventions by detecting early signs of mood disorders and suicide risk. Early detection allows for prompt treatment, which can prevent the progression of symptoms and reduce the risk of suicide.

Personalization: AI can deliver personalized interventions tailored to individual needs and preferences. Personalization enhances treatment adherence and effectiveness, leading to better outcomes for individuals with mood disorders.

Scalability: AI solutions can be scaled to reach large populations, providing support to individuals across diverse settings. Digital therapeutics and AI-powered monitoring tools can reduce the need for frequent in-person appointments, lowering overall treatment costs.

Conclusion

AI has the potential to revolutionize the diagnosis, treatment, and prevention of mood disorders and suicide. By leveraging AI technology, mental health care can become more accessible, timely, and personalized. However, the deployment of AI in this field must be guided by ethical considerations and evidence-based practices to ensure safety, effectiveness, and user satisfaction. The use of already available smart apps should be done cautiously, and professional consultation is always recommended for informed decision and timely intervention. Given the current challenges, it is recommended that AI be used as a complement to existing clinical practices in managing Mood disorders rather than as the primary decision-maker. This approach suggests that AI should support the psychiatrist-patient relationship by facilitating

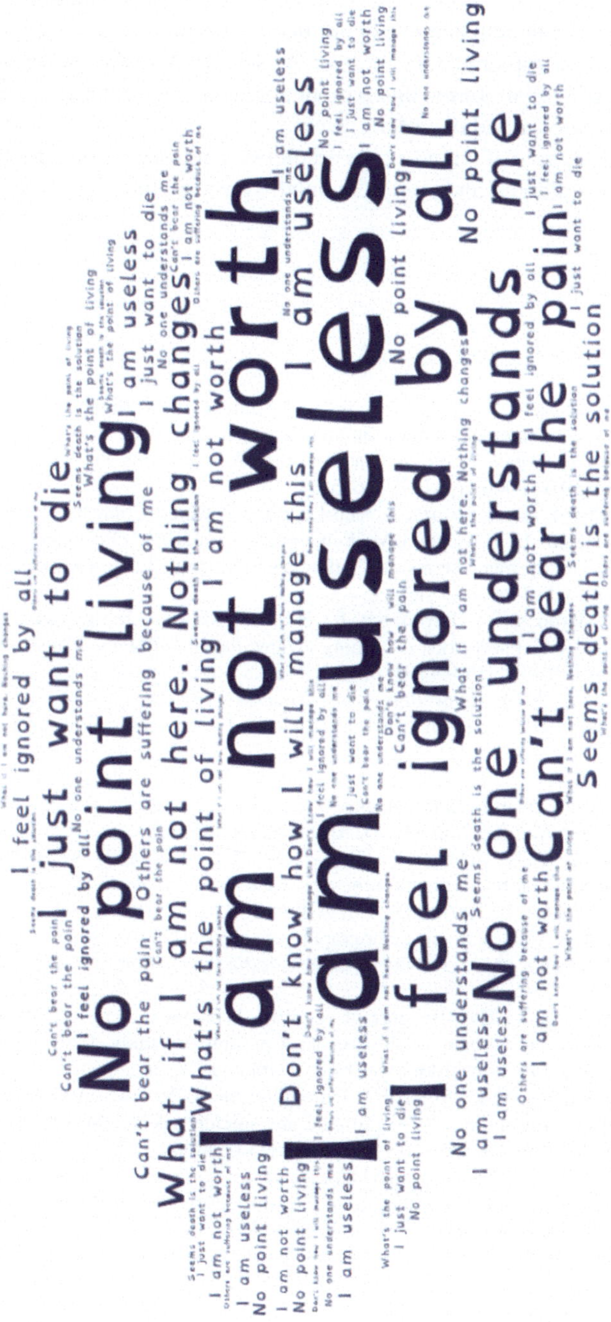

Fig. 6.2 Pictorial sample of how sentiment rich words are analysed for their frequency of use

communication and providing supplementary insights, rather than replacing the critical human element in diagnosis and treatment. By focusing on enhancing interaction and understanding, AI can help achieve better healthcare outcomes for patients with mood disorders. This complementary role for AI sets the foundation for designing systems that prioritize collaboration and patient engagement, which are essential for effective management of mood disorders.

There is a promising role of AI in suicide prediction and intervention; however, the data base need to be enlarged and complemented with real clinical data for credible accuracy.

References

Aldhyani, T. H. H., Alsubari, S. N., Alshebami, A. S., Alkahtani, H., & Ahmed, Z. A. T. (2022). Detecting and analyzing suicidal ideation on social media using deep learning and machine learning models. *International Journal of Environmental Research and Public Health, 19*(19), 12635. https://doi.org/10.3390/ijerph191912635

Benrimoh, D. *et al.* (2018). *Aifred Health*, a Deep Learning Powered Clinical Decision Support System for Mental Health. In: S. Escalera, M. Weimer (Eds.) *The NIPS '17 competition: Building intelligent systems*. The Springer Series on Challenges in Machine Learning. Springer. https://doi.org/10.1007/978-3-319-94042-7_13

Castillo-Sánchez, G., Marques, G., Dorronzoro, E., et al. (2020). Suicide risk assessment using machine learning and social networks: A scoping review. *Journal of Medical Systems, 44*(205), 1. https://doi.org/10.1007/s10916-020-01669-5

Cerrato, P., & Halamka, J. (2020). *Reinventing clinical decision support: Data analytics, artificial intelligence, and diagnostic reasoning* (1st Ed.). Taylor & Francis. https://doi.org/10.1201/978 1003034339

Cheng, Q., Li, T. M., Kwok, C. L., Zhu, T., & Yip, P. S. (2017). Assessing Suicide Risk and Emotional Distress in Chinese Social Media: A Text Mining and Machine Learning Study. *Journal of Medical Internet Research, 19*(7), Article e243. https://doi.org/10.2196/jmir.7276

Graham, S., Depp, C., Lee, E. E., Nebeker, C., Tu, X., Kim, H. C., & Jeste, D. V. (2019). Artificial intelligence for mental health and mental illnesses: An overview. *Current Psychiatry Reports, 21*(11), 116. https://doi.org/10.1007/s11920-019-1094-0

Halder, S., & Mahato, A. K. (2016). Socio-demographic and clinical characteristics of patients who attempt suicide: A hospital-based study from Eastern India. *East Asian Archives of Psychiatry, 26*(3), 98–103.

Halder, S., & Mahato, A. K. (2024). Benefits of cognitive behavior therapy with neuroscience-informed psychoeducation in young adult patients: A preliminary study. *Taiwanese Journal of Psychiatry, 38*(3), 142–146. https://doi.org/10.4103/TPSY.TPSY_26_24

Hua, L. L., Lee, J., Rahmandar, M. H., Sigel, E. J., Committee on Adolescence, & Council on Injury, Violence, and Poison Prevention. (2024). Suicide and suicide risk in adolescents. *Pediatrics, 153*(1), e2023064800. https://doi.org/10.1542/peds.2023-064800

Institute of Health Metrics and Evaluation (IHME). (n.d.). *Global health data exchange (GHDx)*. Retrieved November 19, 2024, from http://ghdx.healthdata.org/gbd-results-tool?params=gbd-api-2019-permalink/27a7644e8ad28e739382d31e77589dd7.

Kerkhof, A. J., & Arensman, E. (2000). Attempted suicide and deliberate self-harm: Epidemiology and risk factors. In M. G. Gelder, J. J. López-Ibor, & A. Nancy (Eds.), *New Oxford textbook of psychiatry* (4.15.2). Oxford University Press.

Lekkas, D., & Jacobson, N. C. (2023). The hidden depths of suicidal discourse: Network analysis and natural language processing unmask uncensored expression. *Digital Health, 9*, 20552076231210710. https://doi.org/10.1177/20552076231210714
Levkovich, I., & Elyoseph, Z. (2023). Identifying depression and its determinants upon initiating treatment: ChatGPT versus primary care physicians. *Family Medicine and Community Health, 11*(4), Article e002391. https://doi.org/10.1136/fmch-2023-002391
Mitchell, A. J., Rao, S., & Vaze, A. (2011). International comparison of clinicians' ability to identify depression in primary care: meta-analysis and meta-regression of predictors. *The British journal of general practice: the journal of the Royal College of General Practitioners, 61*(583), e72–e80.
Nock, M. K., Hwang, I., Sampson, N. A., & Kessler, R. C. (2010). Mental disorders, comorbidity and suicidal behavior: Results from the National Comorbidity Survey Replication. *Molecular Psychiatry, 15*(8), 868–876. https://doi.org/10.1038/mp.2009.29
Park, C. H. K., Lee, J. W., Lee, S. Y., Moon, J., Jeon, D. W., Shim, S. H., Cho, S. J., Kim, S. G., Lee, J., Paik, J. W., Kim, M. H., You, S., Jeon, H. J., Rhee, S. J., Kim, M. J., Kim, J., & Ahn, Y. M. (2020). Suicide risk factors across suicidal ideators, single suicide attempters, and multiple suicide attempters. *Journal of Psychiatric Research, 131*, 1–8. https://doi.org/10.1016/j.jpsychires.2020.08.018
Posner, K., Oquendo, M. A., Gould, M., Stanley, B., & Davies, M. (2007). Columbia classification algorithm of suicide assessment (C-CASA): Classification of suicidal events in the FDA's pediatric suicidal risk analysis of antidepressants. *The American Journal of Psychiatry, 164*(7), 1035–1043. https://doi.org/10.1176/ajp.2007.164.7.1035
Ramírez-Cifuentes, D., Freire, A., Baeza-Yates, R., Puntí, J., Medina-Bravo, P., Velazquez, D. A., Gonfaus, J. M., & Gonzàlez, J. (2020). Detection of Suicidal Ideation on Social Media: Multimodal, Relational, and Behavioral Analysis. *Journal of Medical Internet Research, 22*(7), Article e17758. https://doi.org/10.2196/17758
Suominen, K., Haukka, J., Valtonen, H. M., & Lönnqvist, J. (2009). Outcome of patients with major depressive disorder after serious suicide attempt. *The Journal of Clinical Psychiatry, 70*(10), 1372–1378. https://doi.org/10.4088/JCP.09m05110blu
Tadesse, M. M., Lin, H., Xu, B., & Yang, L. (2020). Detection of suicide ideation in social media forums using deep learning. *Algorithms, 13*(1), 7. https://doi.org/10.3390/a13010007
Yeskuatov, E., Chua, S. L., & Foo, L. K. (2022). Leveraging Reddit for Suicidal Ideation Detection: A Review of Machine Learning and Natural Language Processing Techniques. *International Journal of Environmental Research and Public Health, 19*(16), 10347. https://doi.org/10.3390/ijerph191610347

Chapter 7
Schizophrenia and Related Psychosis

Abstract Schizophrenia is undoubtedly the most intriguing as well as disabling mental ill health condition. The vividity of its symptoms across diagnosed patients which is somehow due to unique psychosocial and biological predisposition of the individual makes schizophrenia a complex illness to understand. The present chapter gives a brief background about schizophrenia, and how Artificial Intelligence (AI) may be used in its management. We discuss the use of AI in its diagnosis, including implications in the prodrome phase. Further specific implications in terms of AI-augmented psychoeducation, cognitive retraining and role in relapse prevention are discussed.

Keywords Psychosis · Schizophrenia · Cognitive training · AI-augmented psychoeducation

Overview

Schizophrenia is known as the paradigmatic illness of psychiatry. Psychosis and schizophrenia at times are used interchangeably but are not the same. Psychosis is predominantly a set of psychopathological symptoms, which is predominantly present and considered a hallmark of schizophrenia and characterized by disordered thinking, often accompanied by delusions or hallucinations. Psychosis is not confined to schizophrenia only and could be seen in several other disorders including brief psychotic disorder, delusional disorder, schizophreniform disorder, mood disorders when in severe form, substance use disorders and personality disorders. It may result from medical or neurologic conditions also.

Schizophrenia is a complicated and varied condition that is sometimes referred to as a "group of schizophrenias". It is becoming more widely acknowledged for a number of different illnesses with similar neurological correlations and symptoms. Conventionally, schizophrenia has been classified into Paranoid, Hebephrenic or Disorganized, Catatonic, Undifferentiated and Residual subtypes. However, the subtypes had little relevance in terms of research, and often symptoms overlapped,

S. Halder et al., *Navigating AI in Mental Health Care*,
https://doi.org/10.1007/978-981-96-9744-1_7

and subsequently the new edition of the classificatory systems, both ICD 11 and DSM 5, no longer list the subtypes. These updates are based on consensus recommendations of the concerned public bodies and meant for uniformity in the classification as well as to keep the classification description at par with changing psychosocial, cultural as well as scientific perspectives. However, it also denotes the enigma behind mental illness, especially about their cause.

What Causes Schizophrenia: The etiological theories of schizophrenia point towards heterogeneous risk factors. Genetic predisposition makes an individual more prone to develop schizophrenia; individual imbalances and deformities in the brain physiology and chemistry, combined with stress factors, increase the risk of developing schizophrenia manyfold.

The complex interaction between a number of endogenous and exogenous elements that affect neurodevelopment of an individual appears to be the cause of the illness. Because of this intricacy, it is too simplistic to classify schizophrenia based on linear connections between a small number of biomarkers or to attribute it to single-cause mechanisms. The mechanisms underlying the onset, relapse, symptomatology, cognitive deficits, and treatment of schizophrenia remain elusive despite years of research using traditional statistical and machine learning (ML) approaches, likely due to a lack of appropriate analytical tools to address the multifaceted nature of the condition.

How Prevalent the Condition is: Lifetime prevalence of psychotic disorders varies widely across studies, primarily due to methodological differences. Schizophrenia affects approximately 24 million people or 1 in 300 people (0.32%) worldwide. This rate is 1 in 222 people (0.45%) among adults (IHME). Some other national surveys reflect a slightly different percentage for lifetime prevalence of schizophrenia, e.g. 1.25% in China (Chang et al., 2017); 2.3% for community-dwelling adult population in Singapore (Subramaniam et al., 2021). The estimated lifetime prevalence of schizophrenia and schizophreniform disorder in community epidemiological surveys using fully structured lay-administered diagnostic interviews have been in the range 0.3–1.6% (Bland, 1988; Canino et al., 1987; Hwu et al., 1989; Keith & Matthews, 1991; Wittchen et al., 1992). But irrespective of these small variances, schizophrenia remains a complex disorder to understand.

Progression of Schizophrenia: The heterogeneity of the causal factors and vividity of its symptoms make schizophrenia a complex diagnosis. The typical age of onset for schizophrenia is in late adolescence or early twenties, with a slightly later onset in females (Häfner et al., 1994). It is another disturbing fact that more than two out of three people with psychosis in the world do not receive specialist mental health care.

Schizophrenia typically follows a prodromal phase with less schizophrenia-like symptoms. Approximately 30% of patients in the prodromal phase progress to psychosis within a 3-year follow-up period. The prodromal phase varies for different individuals and is becoming an important intervention domain. It is a common observation that there is a significant time gap between the first observable set of symptoms and treatment sought in patients with schizophrenia (Loebel et al., 1992). It is also well established that the duration of illness before treatment is significantly associated with treatment outcome both in terms of time for remission and with level of remission (Craig et al., 2000; Ho et al., 2000). This highlights the importance of identifying people at risk of developing schizophrenia as early as possible. The DSM in its latest revision, i.e. DSM5 (TR) added Attenuated Psychosis (APS) as one of the conditions for further study. It is a syndrome also referred to as clinical high-risk state, at-risk mental state, or ultra-high-risk state, referring to symptoms that are psychotic in nature but below the threshold for consideration as counting towards the diagnosis of a psychotic disorder. The symptoms are usually less severe and more transient and individuals with APS may later meet diagnostic criteria for schizophrenia, bipolar disorder, or another disorder with psychosis.

AI in Schizophrenia Diagnosis

Diagnosing schizophrenia could be an easy task for a trained professional. However, as said earlier, co-morbidity is a rule rather than an exception; the task becomes difficult if affective or mood symptoms overlap with schizophrenic illness.

Schizophrenia typically follows a prodromal phase with less schizophrenia-like symptoms. Approximately 30% of patients in the prodromal phase progress to psychosis within a 3-year follow-up period. Artificial intelligence systems can anticipate the likelihood of conversion and relapse, allowing for timely treatments. Artificial Neural Network (ANN) models have been used to predict psychosis based on the lack of content and the mention of voices in speech samples. Some researchers have employed artificial intelligence algorithms on massive electronic health records (EHRs) to predict the onset of schizophrenia, with excellent results. One of the most promising applications of AI in schizophrenia care is in the area of diagnosis. Schizophrenia is a complex condition that can be difficult to diagnose early, especially since its symptoms often overlap with those of other mental health disorders. AI systems, however, are capable of processing and analysing vast amounts of data, such as genetic information, brain scans, and medical records. By identifying patterns and correlations that might be missed by human analysis, AI can help predict the likelihood of an individual developing schizophrenia, particularly if there is a hereditary predisposition. Early detection is crucial in schizophrenia management, as it allows for the timely initiation of treatment, which can prevent the progression of the disorder and mitigate the severity of symptoms. AI's ability to predict the onset of schizophrenia before symptoms become pronounced could revolutionize the approach to mental health care, enabling preventative measures and early interventions that could change the course of the disease. Machine learning algorithms have been employed to distinguish individuals with schizophrenia from healthy controls by analysing variations in grey and white matter, including differences in size and density, with remarkable precision. Functional Magnetic Resonance Imaging (fMRI) data has provided insights into the neural networks of schizophrenia patients, revealing that they tend to activate a less distinct set of brain regions compared to healthy individuals. AI has also been applied to Electroencephalogram (EEG) scans to predict the onset of psychosis with accuracy rates ranging from 74 to 93%. Beyond neuroimaging, AI techniques have explored facial features for early detection of schizophrenia, utilizing tools like eye-tracking and analysis of facial expressions. Communication abilities, such as handwriting patterns and keyword usage on social media, have also been analysed through AI to detect schizophrenia. Additionally, AI has been used to assess the risk of schizophrenia in healthy first-degree relatives, offering a proactive approach to identifying those who may be predisposed to the disorder.

Recent advances in deep learning—a subfield of ML—have provided the field of neuropsychiatry with powerful tools to model and analyse complex, high-dimensional, and nonlinear problems. Deep learning, a subtype of machine learning, uses deep neural networks (DNNs), which are algorithms inspired by the human nervous system and made up of numerous interconnected layers of nonlinear processing units known as artificial neurons. During training, DNNs modify the strengths (weights) of neuron connections, similar to how the nervous system learns.

One significant distinction between deep learning and classic machine learning systems is the type of data they handle. Traditional machine learning methods, such as support vector machines (SVMs), decision trees, and random forests, as well as statistical methods like multivariate regression, are often used on highly processed data. These methods employ a small number of features retrieved from high-dimensional raw data, with the premise that these features are important to a certain job (for example, power ratios between electroencephalography [EEG] frequency bands). In contrast, DNNs can process high-dimensional raw or slightly processed data and automatically learn to extract the most relevant characteristics for a given task. This ability to work with unstructured data and uncover complex, nonlinear relationships is critical to deep learning's superior performance in tasks such as diagnosing schizophrenia using simultaneous EEG and functional magnetic resonance imaging (fMRI) data or predicting patient prognosis based on electrophysiological data. In contrast, DNNs can process high-dimensional raw or barely processed data and automatically learn to extract the most relevant characteristics for a task. This ability to work with unstructured data and uncover complex, nonlinear relationships is critical to deep learning's superior performance in tasks such as diagnosing schizophrenia using simultaneous EEG and functional magnetic resonance imaging (fMRI) data or predicting patient prognosis based on electrophysiological data. Although the conceptual basis for DNNs have been developed for decades, recent technological advances—such as the availability of powerful processors (GPUs), enormous electronic datasets, and algorithmic innovations—have resulted in broad acceptance and development of DNN technology. This progress has enabled discoveries that seemed impossible just a few years before. While DNNs have the potential to improve diagnosis, subtyping, and treatment decisions for schizophrenia, their function in furthering our understanding of the disorder's underlying causes is unclear. DNNs are frequently referred to as "black-box" models because the nonlinear transformations and high-dimensional representations they employ to solve problems are too sophisticated to be easily understood. Unlike regression models, whose coefficients provide interpretable information about the relationship between inputs and outputs, DNN models do not provide direct insights into the internal mechanics of the issues they solve. However, the view of DNNs as impenetrable is being challenged by the development of explainable AI techniques, which seek to discover the inputs most relevant to a model's output after a prediction has been made. Furthermore, researchers are beginning to provide DNNs with cause-and-effect models (hypotheses) of reality, which could lead to novel mechanical explanations for schizophrenia.

Identifying Individuals in Prodrome Phase: The consultation pattern of caregivers for patients with schizophrenia suggests that patients are usually brought for consultation mostly in the acute phase, rather than in the prodrome stage, thus almost negating the clinical relevance of the prodromal phase. However, a thorough assessment of the prodromal phase can reduce relapse risks and better treatment outcomes for patients with schizophrenia and related psychosis. However, early diagnosis or identifying individuals in their prodromal phase could be less easy than said. The concept of prodrome is poorly defined and professionals are not uniform on defining or the treatment guidelines for prodrome. This is primarily due to lack of confirmed biomarkers which can uniformly diagnose schizophrenia across all populations. In addition, individuals in the prodromal phase may develop different sets of symptoms in the acute phase, warranting a different approach for treatment. The conceptualization of prodrome has undergone several changes, as we see in the 3rd revised edition of the DSM, prodromal features of schizophrenia were listed and provide an operationalized criteria of nine symptoms for schizophrenia prodrome as follows:

1. Marked social isolation or withdrawal
2. Marked impairment in role functioning
3. Markedly peculiar behaviour
4. Marked impairment in personal hygiene and grooming
5. Blunted or inappropriate affect
6. Digressive, vague, over-elaborate or circumstantial speech, or poverty of speech, or poverty of content of speech
7. Odd beliefs or magical thinking
8. Unusual perceptual experiences
9. Marked lack of initiative, interests, or energy.

However, this list of criteria has been dropped from the DSM-IV. While clinical history and clinical interview are essentially required to make an impression of prodrome; reliable information is often not available from caregivers.

Case Example: Mr J is a 21-year-old postgraduate student, pursuing MBA. He was referred to the institute's counselling centre after poor academic performance in the semester examination, and his faculty mentor doubted J being "depressed". Upon interviewing, J denied feeling depressed and mentioned he fails to connect with people in his class in general and attends class just because his parents wanted him to pursue the program. Further enquiry revealed, he hardly had any close friends. He was often mocked by his classmates for wearing the same clothes consecutively for several days. His mentor faculty reported, he was often found preoccupied and staring at blank during lectures. He was very regular to class though. Unlike other students who would react strongly or make excuses if scolded on certain issues, J would be quietly listening, as if nothing happened. The counsellor called his parents to have a word, who mentioned, J was of quiet nature since childhood, and did not interact much even within familial circle or neighbourhood. He had a peculiar habit of keeping sugar in his room to feed ants, as he believed they were from the underworld. While this led to frequent tiffs with his mother, they never gave much importance to these. His parents did not like the advice to consult J with a mental health professional for any possible intervention required. After around 6 months, J's faculty mentor reported he had left the programme and was under psychiatric treatment possibly diagnosed with schizophrenia.

Cases like J are common and it reflects a generic mentality of avoiding mental health intervention, particularly if it is pharmacotherapy, unless there are very evident symptoms causing discomfort, danger to the patient or family members. However, it costs in terms of loss of opportunity of possible prevention of the acute psychotic phase like J had. It also costs in terms of how long J would take to reach his premorbid level, if at all he would reach the premorbid level or how nearer he would reach the premorbid level.

Whether AI Is Implied in Such a Situation: There is emerging literature on use of AI in detection of schizophrenia and how patients with schizophrenia can be differentiated from healthy controls. However, much of this AI application is relatable to stage when symptoms are florid, or at most when individuals can be said to have ultra-high risk and AI assists in clinical decision-making. But can AI be stretched further to give a much earlier prediction? It might be a difficult question to answer. The current understanding of schizophrenia aetiology is multifactorial and reflects an interaction between genetic vulnerability and environmental contributors and risk factors such as pregnancy and birth complications, childhood trauma, migration, social isolation, urbanicity, and substance abuse, alone and in combination, acting at a number of levels over time, influence the individual's likelihood to develop the disorder. Can these risk factors be tapped in quantifiable data? The data for predictive utility of AI in schizophrenia comes primarily from imaging and scans as well as blood-based diagnostics. The literature is definitely promising but yet not conclusive. Very recent research claims of being successful in identifying biomarkers that were predictive of high hallucinations and of high delusions states, and of future psychiatric hospitalizations related to them, more so when personalized by gender and diagnosis (Hill et al., 2024). Several others highlight the role of increased levels of glutamate (Galińska-Skok & Waszkiewicz, 2022; Lai et al., 2016). Similarly those focussing on neurostructural biomarkers highlight grey matter volume reductions in high-risk patients compared with healthy controls in hippocampal/parahippocampal areas, cingulate cortex, medial and lateral frontal cortex and medial parietal cortex. Also, the high-risk subjects with later transition to psychosis show larger pituitary volumes than subjects without later psychosis (Galińska-Skok & Waszkiewicz, 2022). However, these clinical data are yet too small for conclusive inference by AI. Researchers also highlight other set of biomarkers that included neuropsychological, stop-signal, saccadic/eye control as well as auditory stimulation paradigms in individuals diagnosed with schizophrenia, schizoaffective disorder and bipolar disorder with accompanying psychosis, and could identify three neurobiologically distinct psychosis biotypes, characterized by poor cognitive and sensorimotor functions; moderate cognitive dysfunction and sensorimotor hyper-reactivity; and almost normal cognitive and sensorimotor functions (Clementz et al., 2015). This might be early to comment, but there is a scope of combining all these datasets for a better prediction model. There are counter views too on early identification of schizophrenia in people at risk, suggesting screening all genetically vulnerable persons in the general population has no consequences for treatment. It advises early diagnosis by psychiatrists but recommends larger groups and longer studies in order to demonstrate conclusively the preventive effect of interventions prior to a first psychosis (Klaassen et al., 2006). Others suggest prediction of transitions from at risk to psychosis could be improved by a stronger weighting of certain early symptoms and by introducing neurocognitive tests into a stepwise risk assessment (Riecher-Rössler et al., 2009). Irrespective of the current status, there is no denial that prevention is always better than cure.

Use of AI in Management of Schizophrenia and Related Conditions

AI-augmented Psychoeducation: Compared to diagnostic utility, implication of AI might be relatively better in management from different perspectives. One of the very basic approaches in management of schizophrenia includes **psychoeducation**, which is universal for most clinical conditions. A standard psychoeducation includes explaining signs and symptoms of the illness, its aetiology, and standard approach of treatment, which is targeted to improve treatment compliance, reduce stigma as well as care burden of family members. However, with use of AI, the psychoeducation model can be made more customized and personal to the client. There are emerging new models of psychoeducation which recommend incorporating a neuropsychological explanation of the condition as well as the psychotherapeutic process (Ekhtiari et al., 2017; Halder & Mahato, 2024). The models have further scope of embedding with AI, where personal clinical information, e.g. brain scans, blood-based diagnostics may be added to provide a comprehensive psychoeducation which can also include possible risks of relapse, as well as treatment outcome (Table 7.1).

Further, patients with schizophrenia have varied outcomes depending on their genetic predisposition, symptom type, age of onset, severity, comorbid conditions, and psychosocial support to name a few. It is a known fact that all individuals with schizophrenia do not respond equally to the same group of medications. A biomarker-based profiling by an AI algorithm can help in deciding the best possible combination of antipsychotics and other medications required and thus very much personalizing the treatment for the patient. Patients with schizophrenia often struggle to adhere to the medication regime and risk relapse. AI-based applications can help track medicine usage patterns of the patient for triggering alerts during vulnerable periods

Table 7.1 Conventional psychoeducation augmented with AI component

Conventional psychoeducation	Additional components with AI
• Sign and Symptoms of illness • Nature and course of illness • Treatment requirements and modalities • Relapse- risk and prediction	Neuropsychological explanation of the condition as well as therapy process + Analysis of clinical data (brain scan, blood-based diagnostic test) and profiling + Identification of individual risk factors + Better prognosis estimate

so that doses are not missed. AI can also devise personalized daily activity charts for patients as per their treatment needs, including reminders for taking medicines. In the event, patients miss any of their activities in the schedule, which is a common phenomenon, it may advise the patient for further needful and remove a state of confusion deciding what to do next. As patients with schizophrenia actively need supportive therapy, AI-based chatbots or virtual therapists can do a great deal in assisting them in real-life situations.

Cognitive Training: In recent years cognitive retraining has gained prominence in comprehensive management of schizophrenia. Cognitive retraining is not for symptomatic relief but primarily targets improvement in daily functionality of patients with schizophrenia by targeting cognitive functions. While the early models of cognitive training started with paper–pencil-based tests, they gradually got upgraded to computer based models and now await further upgrade by embedding them with AI.

Case Study

Vinit (name changed) is a 46-year-old male, married, working as an IT professional, who was diagnosed with schizophrenia 10 years back. He lost his job about 5 years back due to his symptoms interfering with occupational output, as he suspected on his colleagues, missed deadlines frequently and even those completed on time were not up to the mark.

He has been under medications and psychotherapeutic intervention. The psychologist considered his cognitive impairment, which were evident in the domains of attention, memory and executive functioning. Thus, apart from supportive psychotherapy, cognitive retraining was also included in the management plan to improve daily living functioning.

A conventional model of cognitive training (Fig. 7.1) for Vinit targeting his cognitive skills typically looks like the following:

The conventional cognitive training models using the paper–pencil-based tasks are definitely effective and pretty suitable where computerized versions are not feasible. They also demand a certain level of customization depending on the educational

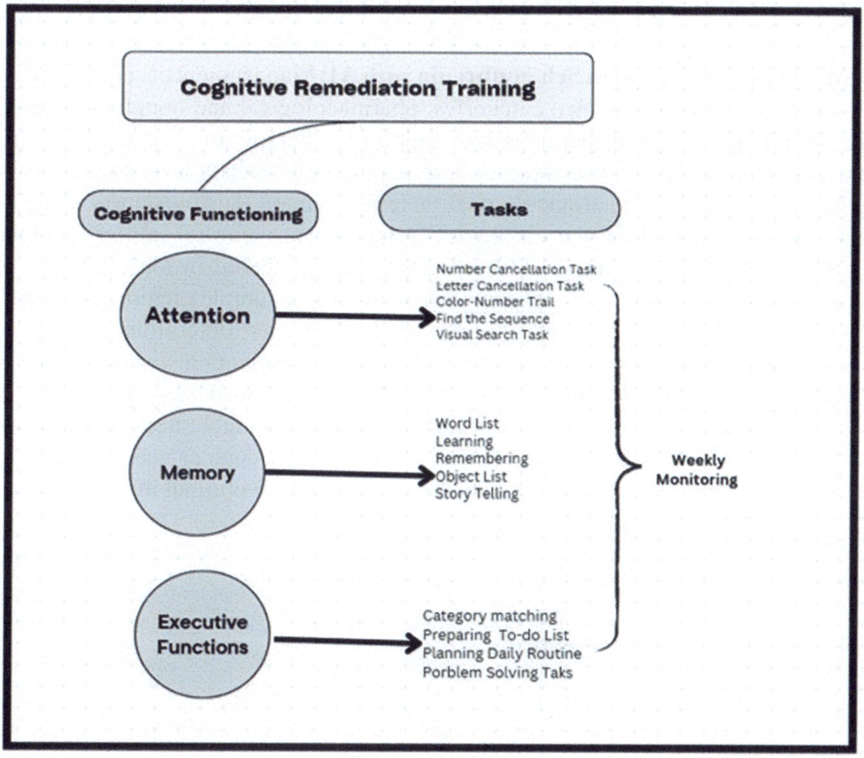

Fig. 7.1 Conventional model of cognitive training

and cultural background of the individuals for enhanced effectiveness. The models, while effective, do require regular and continuous engagement and monitoring for changing difficulty levels of the task upon its masterly. There also had been a need of devising these training tasks more relatable to daily life functioning, as the transfer of learning through mastery on cognitive tasks to real-life circumstances was doubted. The computerized versions did a better job in terms of devising these tasks in the form of games, but there was still much left.

AI-embed cognitive training models hold a certain edge over conventional models. While they will definitely be effective like the conventional ones, there is a much larger scope of customization, due to their inherent capacity to learn on its own the baseline capacities of the patient. Accordingly, cognitive training games can be tailored to enhance diverse cognitive abilities of patients (Fig. 7.2). By using adaptive algorithms, these games customize training plans by analysing user performance in real-time, dynamically adjusting difficulty levels and delivering targeted exercises for optimal improvement, whereas cognitive training programmes prepared by clinician and delivered in clinic set-up are less flexible, time bound as per schedule of therapist, and less relatable to real-life situations. The AI-based models can give comparative feedback of the patient across timeline to see improvement in desired cognitive domain.

Enhancing Treatment in Schizophrenia with AI: Management of schizophrenia is frequently classified into two categories: pharmacological and nonpharmacological. Nonpharmacological therapies like supportive therapy are intended to assist patients in coping with their symptoms and maintaining a steady level of psychosocial functioning. While pharmacological therapies remain the foundation of treatment, they are founded on neurobiological principles of neurotransmitter reuptake and release. Beyond diagnosis, AI holds significant potential in the treatment of schizophrenia. Managing schizophrenia often involves a complex regimen of medications, tailored to each patient's unique needs. However, determining the most effective medication and dosage can be challenging, as patients respond differently to treatments, and the risk of side effects is always present. AI can address these challenges by analysing patient data to identify the most suitable treatment options (Fig. 7.3). AI-driven systems can evaluate various factors, such as genetic markers, patient history, and real-time health data, to recommend the optimal medication and

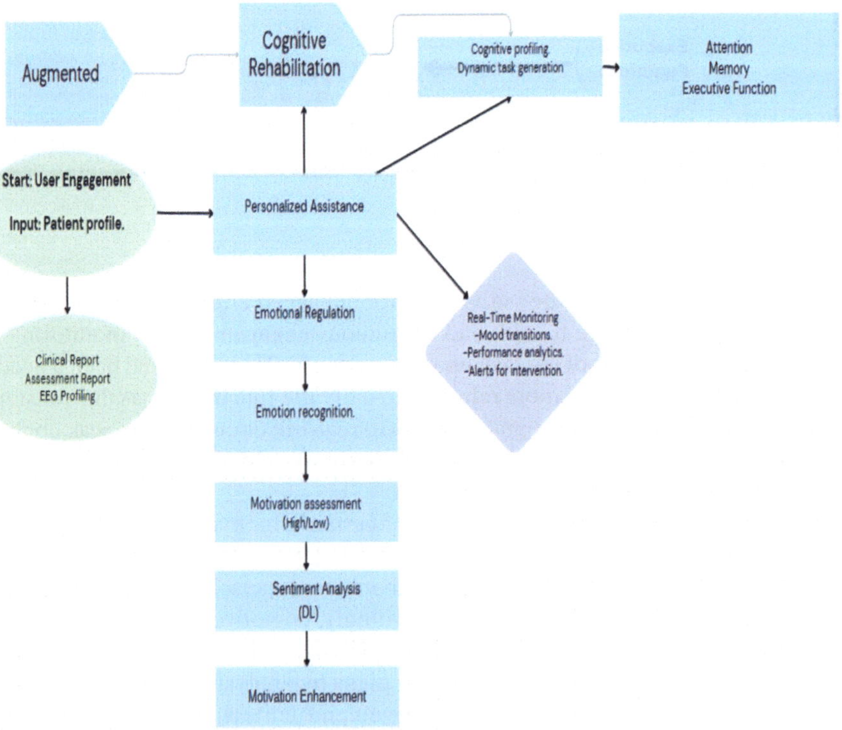

Fig. 7.2 AI-driven model for cognitive training

dosage for each individual. This personalized approach not only enhances the efficacy of treatment but also reduces the likelihood of adverse effects. Furthermore, AI can continuously monitor a patient's response to treatment, allowing healthcare providers to adjust medications as needed to ensure the best possible outcomes. AI plays a varied function in therapy, ranging from helping medication research and development to personalising therapeutic interventions. AI algorithms can use genetic, environmental, and clinical data to predict individual reactions to certain medications, paving the way for personalized medicine in schizophrenia therapy. This not only improves therapeutic efficacy but also reduces unwanted effects, resulting in better patient outcomes and quality of life. In addition, artificial intelligence has the potential to greatly improve long-term schizophrenia management efforts. AI-powered smartphone apps and wearable devices provide new avenues for continuous symptom monitoring and treatment adherence, allowing for more rapid interventions and improved illness management. Predictive analytics can help identify possible relapses or worsening, allowing for preventive care options.

AI can have further specific use when dealing with psychotic features in individuals with schizophrenia in recovery phase. Virtual reality (VR) and avatars are examples of AI tools that are helping patients cope with the voices, technically called hallucinations they hear. By enabling users to "talk" to the voices in their heads, these avatars help people feel better and manage hallucinations. People who don't react well to conventional treatments have found that VR therapy improves their mood, lessens hallucinations, and improves their quality of life.

AI in Medication Management and Patient Monitoring: Another critical aspect of schizophrenia care is medication management, which is essential for preventing relapses and maintaining stability in patients. AI can play a pivotal role in helping

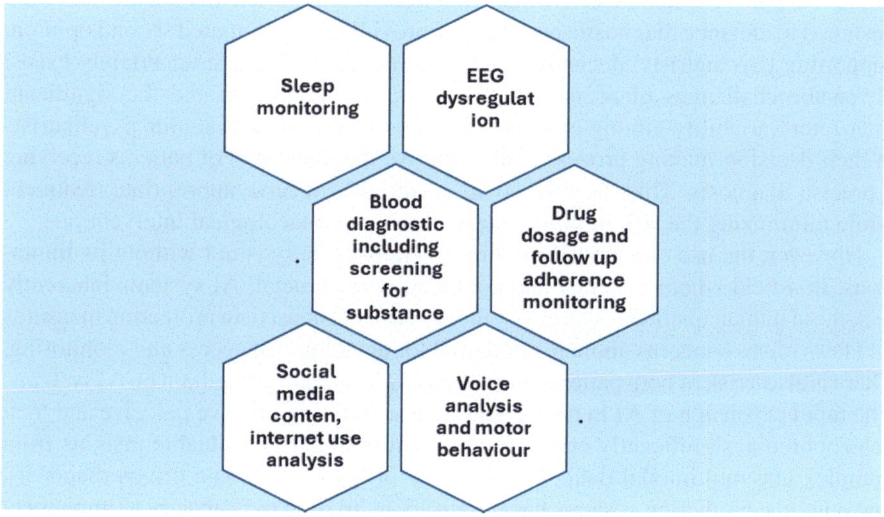

Fig. 7.3 AI implications in schizophrenia

patients adhere to their treatment plans. For example, AI-powered applications can remind patients to take their medications, monitor their adherence, and alert healthcare providers if a patient is at risk of missing doses or experiencing side effects. AI can predict how well a treatment might work for a person by analysing genetic data and brain scans, and robots are also being used in therapy. This aids medical professionals in developing more individualized treatment programmes that are more effective for each patient. In order to provide assistance more quickly and efficiently, AI is even assisting physicians in determining whether patients are taking their prescriptions as prescribed and predicting the likelihood of aggressive behaviour.

Additionally, AI can be used to develop predictive models that foresee potential relapses based on behavioural and health data. By identifying early warning signs, AI systems can prompt timely interventions, such as adjusting medication or increasing patient support, to prevent a full-blown relapse. This proactive approach can significantly improve long-term outcomes for individuals living with schizophrenia. All things considered, AI is improving the intelligence and individual needs-focused nature of schizophrenia treatment, giving those who suffer from the illness hope for a brighter future.

Advancing Our Understanding of Schizophrenia: AI is not only beneficial for individual patient care but also for advancing our overall understanding of schizophrenia. The ability of AI to analyse large datasets allows researchers to uncover new insights into the underlying mechanisms of the disorder. This could lead to the discovery of novel biomarkers, improved diagnostic criteria, and the development of more effective treatments. AI's capacity to integrate and analyse diverse types of data, from genetic information to neuroimaging, enables a more holistic understanding of schizophrenia. This comprehensive approach may help to unravel the complexities of the disorder, leading to better-targeted therapies and ultimately, improved patient outcomes. Artificial intelligence-supported diagnostic tools are designed to enhance diagnostic accuracy by providing an automated second opinion, supporting psychiatrists' decisions, and assisting in cases where uncertainty exists. Given the challenges of accurately diagnosing schizophrenia and the significant inter-rater variability among experts, a diagnostic algorithm that aids psychiatrists in their decision-making process could improve the likelihood of patients receiving a precise diagnosis. This, in turn, could ensure they receive appropriate treatment while minimizing the risk of unnecessary psychopharmacological interventions.

However, the use of artificial intelligence in psychiatry is not without its limitations. In a field where empathy and compassion are crucial, AI systems inherently lack these human qualities. Moreover, the absence of robust data protection measures and laws raises concerns about the potential for unauthorized access and monitoring. There is also a risk of both patients and doctors becoming overly reliant on AI systems. The rapid expansion of AI in recent years is transforming how we perceive and treat schizophrenia, significantly enhancing our ability to extract valuable insights from complex and multimodal data. The accuracy of automated, data-driven diagnosis, and outcome prediction systems has improved, increasing our capacity to implement preventive or more effective personalized treatment strategies. However, while AI can help alleviate some of the burdens of schizophrenia on patients and caregivers, it also introduces ethical challenges that must be carefully evaluated and addressed. Considering the potential harm that a misdiagnosis or incorrect prediction could inflict on a patient, AI systems must undergo continuous error evaluation and have appropriate protocols in place to protect patient welfare. While the current application of AI in schizophrenia is limited, its future advancements hold significant promise. The hope is that AI systems will be developed to make medical treatment for schizophrenia more efficient and accessible.

Advantages and Limitations of Artificial Intelligence in Schizophrenia: The goal of artificial intelligence-supported diagnostic tools is to improve diagnostic confidence, provide an automated second opinion, confirm a psychiatrist's judgement, and assist with ambiguous cases. Given the difficulty of determining whether schizophrenia is precisely diagnosed, as well as the significant inter-rater disagreement among experts, a diagnostic algorithm that guides psychiatrists in their decision-making could increase the likelihood of patients receiving an accurate diagnosis, and thus receiving adequate treatment and avoiding unnecessary psychopharmacological interventions. Yet, artificial intelligence isn't without its drawbacks. In the realm of psychiatry, where empathy and compassion are critical, artificial intelligence largely lacks them. In the absence of sufficient data protection methods and laws, artificial intelligence systems may serve as a conduit for hacking and unauthorized monitoring. Furthermore, both the patient and the clinician risk becoming overly reliant on artificial intelligence technologies.

Perspectives of Patients on AI-Driven Predictions of Relapses

Schizophrenia, characterized by both positive and negative symptoms, disrupts daily life and significantly reduces the quality of life for those affected. Positive symptoms include hallucinations, delusions, and disorganized thinking, while negative symptoms involve reduced functioning, such as a lack of motivation and the inability to experience pleasure. Managing schizophrenia is challenging, as more than 80% of patients experience a relapse after their first episode, often requiring intensive care. Preventing relapses and detecting early signs of symptom escalation are critical for improving patient outcomes. Historically, relapse prevention has relied on patient self-reporting and clinician observations. However, these methods are often inadequate due to the individualized nature of schizophrenia symptoms. As a result, researchers have turned to advanced technologies, including artificial intelligence (AI), to improve relapse prediction. Early efforts using statistical methods and clinician assessments lacked the granularity needed to accurately predict relapses. Recent approaches have explored using ecological momentary assessments, smartphone passive sensing, and social media data to provide more nuanced insights into patient behaviour and symptoms. For example, a study by Zhou et al. used smartphone data, such as ambient light and sound, to predict relapses, while Barnett et al. employed passive sensor data like GPS and accelerometer readings to detect early warning signs. Birnbaum et al. analysed Facebook posts, focusing on linguistic features and social media activity, to predict periods leading up to hospitalization. These AI-driven methods show promise in identifying early signs of relapse, but they are still in the early stages of development and require further validation. AI has the potential to revolutionize schizophrenia care by improving relapse prediction and fostering collaboration, and it must be carefully designed to respect patient autonomy and support existing social dynamics. Future research should focus on refining these technologies to ensure they are both effective and ethically sound.

Patients with schizophrenia are often concerned about the unpredictability of their condition. Relapses can occur despite adherence to treatment plans, leaving patients feeling vulnerable and uncertain. The introduction of AI in this context offers a new avenue for detecting early signs of relapse, potentially providing patients with the tools they need to manage their symptoms more effectively. AI systems can analyse large amounts of data, such as behavioural patterns from smartphone sensors or social media activity, to identify subtle changes that may signal an impending relapse. However, the use of AI in schizophrenia relapse prevention is met with mixed feelings among patients. On the one hand, there is optimism about the potential of AI to provide more accurate and timely predictions, enabling earlier interventions that could prevent a full-blown relapse. Patients appreciate the idea of having a technological aid that can continuously monitor their condition, potentially catching signs of trouble that might otherwise go unnoticed. This could lead to more personalized care and a greater sense of control over their illness. On the other hand, patients also express concerns about the implications of relying on AI for such a sensitive aspect of their health. A key concern is the lack of human empathy in AI systems. Schizophrenia is a deeply personal and often isolating experience, and patients value the human connection they have with their healthcare providers and support networks. There is a fear that AI could replace or diminish these relationships, leading to a more clinical and less compassionate approach to care. Additionally, patients worry about the potential for overreliance on AI, which could lead to a reduction in their own agency and decision-making power.

Another significant concern is privacy and data security. The idea of AI systems continuously monitoring their behaviour, even with the intent of preventing relapses, can feel intrusive to patients. The potential for data breaches or misuse of personal information adds to their anxiety. Patients want assurances that their data will be handled with the utmost care and that AI systems will be designed with strong protections in place. Despite these concerns, there is also a recognition of the potential benefits that AI could bring to their lives. Many patients see AI as a tool that could complement, rather than replace, the support they receive from their healthcare providers and loved ones. For instance, AI could help facilitate conversations between patients and their support networks by providing objective data that can be discussed and acted upon collaboratively. This could lead to more informed and supportive relationships, enhancing the overall effectiveness of relapse prevention efforts.

Patients with schizophrenia are cautiously optimistic about the use of AI in relapse prevention; they emphasize the need for these technologies to be developed with a deep understanding of their unique challenges and concerns. AI should not only aim to improve predictive accuracy but also to support the human elements of care that are so vital to their well-being. By balancing technological innovation with empathy and respect for patient autonomy, AI could become a valuable ally in the fight against schizophrenia.

Conclusion

The integration of artificial intelligence (AI) in care of schizophrenia has gained significant momentum in recent years, driven by the urgent need and the increasing demand for accessible care. The global mental health burden, exacerbated by different challenges, has underscored the importance of innovative approaches and AI applications have already demonstrated their potential in diagnosis and management of schizophrenia and other psychoses. It is well implicated in symptom monitoring, disease trajectory prediction and providing psychoeducation, delivered through smartphone apps, and digital gaming. Emerging AI-driven interventions, including therapy and chatbots have capability to teach emotional coping strategies and provide communication support. Avatar-based therapy leveraging computer-generated facial imagery, and intelligent animal-like robots can assist individuals diagnosed with the condition in real-time. These advancements represent a promising frontier in digital psychiatry, offering new avenues for personalized, scalable, and engaging mental health care of patients with psychosis.

The incorporation of AI chatbots and related tools not only bridge gaps in access to care but also expand the possibilities for individualized interventions, enabling a more tailored and patient-centric approach. As AI continues to evolve, its applications in schizophrenia management will likely transform the field, fostering innovative treatments, improved outcomes, and a deeper understanding of this complex condition.

References

Bland R. C. (1988). Psychiatric epidemiology. Canadian journal of psychiatry. *Revue canadienne de psychiatrie, 33*(7), 618–625.

Canino, G. J., Bird, H. R., Shrout, P. E., Rubio-Stipec, M., Bravo, M., Martinez, R., Sesman, M., & Guevara, L. M. (1987). The prevalence of specific psychiatric disorders in Puerto Rico. *Archives of general psychiatry, 44*(8), 727–735.

Chang, W. C., Wong, C. S. M., Chen, E. Y. H., Lam, L. C. W., Chan, W. C., Ng, R. M. K., Hung, S. F., Cheung, E. F. C., Sham, P. C., Chiu, H. F. K., Lam, M., Lee, E. H. M., Chiang, T. P., Chan, L. K., Lau, G. K. W., Lee, A. T. C., Leung, G. T. Y., Leung, J. S. Y., Lau, J. T. F., … Bebbington, P. (2017). Lifetime prevalence and correlates of schizophrenia-spectrum, affective, and other non-affective psychotic disorders in the Chinese adult population. *Schizophrenia Bulletin, 43*(6), 1280–1290. https://doi.org/10.1093/schbul/sbx056

Clementz, B. A., Sweeney, J. A., Hamm, J. P., Ivleva, E. I., Ethridge, L. E., Pearlson, G. D., Keshavan, M. S., & Tamminga, C. A. (2016). Identification of distinct psychosis biotypes using brain-based biomarkers. *The American journal of psychiatry, 173*(4), 373–384.

Craig, T. J., Bromet, E. J., Fennig, S., Tanenberg-Karant, M., Lavelle, J., & Galambos, N. (2000). Is there an association between duration of untreated psychosis and 24-month clinical outcome in a first-admission series? *The American Journal of Psychiatry, 157*(1), 60–66. https://doi.org/10.1176/ajp.157.1.60

Ekhtiari, H., Rezapour, T., Aupperle, R. L., & Paulus, M. P. (2017). Neuroscience-informed psychoeducation for addiction medicine: A neurocognitive perspective. *Progress in Brain Research, 235*, 239–264. https://doi.org/10.1016/bs.pbr.2017.08.013

Galińska-Skok, B., & Waszkiewicz, N. (2022). Markers of Schizophrenia—A critical narrative update. *Journal of Clinical Medicine, 11*(14), 3964. https://doi.org/10.3390/jcm11143964

Häfner, H., Maurer, K., Löffler, W., Fätkenheuer, B., an der Heiden, W., Riecher-Rössler, A., Behrens, S., & Gattaz, W. F. (1994). The epidemiology of early schizophrenia. Influence of age and gender on onset and early course. *The British Journal of Psychiatry, Supplement*(23), 29–38.

Halder, S., & Mahato, A. K. (2024). Benefits of cognitive behavior therapy with neuroscience-informed psychoeducation in young adult patients: A preliminary study. *Taiwanese Journal of Psychiatry, 38*(3), 142–146. https://doi.org/10.4103/TPSY.TPSY_26_24

Hill, M. D., Gill, S. S., Le-Niculescu, H., et al. (2024). Precision medicine for psychotic disorders: Objective assessment, risk prediction, and pharmacogenomics. *Molecular Psychiatry, 29*, 1528–1549. https://doi.org/10.1038/s41380-024-02433-8

Ho, B. C., Andreasen, N. C., Flaum, M., Nopoulos, P., & Miller, D. (2000). Untreated initial psychosis: Its relation to quality of life and symptom remission in first-episode schizophrenia. *The American Journal of Psychiatry, 157*(5), 808–815. https://doi.org/10.1176/appi.ajp.157.5.808

Hwu, H.-G., Yeh, E.-K., & Chang, L.-Y. (1989). Prevalence of psychiatric disorders in Taiwan defined by the Chinese Diagnostic Interview Schedule. *Acta Psychiatrica Scandinavica, 79*(2), 136–147.

Keith, S. J., & Matthews, S. M. (1991). The diagnosis of schizophrenia: a review of onset and duration issues. *Schizophrenia Bulletin, 17*(1), 51–67.

Klaassen, M. C., Nieman, D. H., Becker, H. E., & Linszen, D. H. (2006). Wanneer heeft detectie van hoogrisicofactoren voor een eerste psychose zin? [Is there any point in detecting high-risk factors prior to a first psychosis?]. *Tijdschrift Voor Psychiatrie, 48*(6), 467–476.

Lai, C. Y., Scarr, E., Udawela, M., Everall, I., Chen, W. J., & Dean, B. (2016). Biomarkers in schizophrenia: A focus on blood based diagnostics and theranostics. *World Journal of Psychiatry, 6*(1), 102–117. https://doi.org/10.5498/wjp.v6.i1.102

Loebel, A. D., Lieberman, J. A., Alvir, J. M., Mayerhoff, D. I., Geisler, S. H., & Szymanski, S. R. (1992). Duration of psychosis and outcome in first-episode schizophrenia. *The American Journal of Psychiatry, 149*(9), 1183–1188. https://doi.org/10.1176/ajp.149.9.1183

Riecher-Rössler, A., Pflueger, M. O., Aston, J., Borgwardt, S. J., Brewer, W. J., Gschwandtner, U., & Stieglitz, R. D. (2009). Efficacy of using cognitive status in predicting psychosis: A 7-year follow-up. *Biological Psychiatry, 66*(11), 1023–1030. https://doi.org/10.1016/j.biopsych.2009.07.020

Subramaniam, M., Abdin, E., Vaingankar, J. A., Sambasivam, R., Zhang, Y. J., Shafie, S., Basu, S., Chan, C. T., Tan, C. S., Verma, S. K., Tang, C., Chua, H. C., Heng, D., & Chong, S. A. (2021). Lifetime prevalence and correlates of schizophrenia and other psychotic disorders in Singapore. *Frontiers in Psychiatry, 12*, Article 650674. https://doi.org/10.3389/fpsyt.2021.650674

Wittchen, H. U., Essau, C. A., von Zerssen, D., Krieg, J. C., & Zaudig, M. (1992). Lifetime and six-month prevalence of mental disorders in the Munich Follow-Up Study. *European Archives of Psychiatry and Clinical Neuroscience, 241*(4), 247–258.

Chapter 8
Childhood and Adolescent Disorders

Abstract Just like adults, children and adolescents too face mental health issues. Recent advancements in artificial intelligence (AI) imply exciting potential for its application in paediatric healthcare. This is especially true for early detection of developmental issues, like autism and intellectual disability, where timely intervention is critical. As availability of trained professionals is an issue globally; technology, particularly those which utilize AI has the potential to significantly enhance mental health services, acting as a workforce multiplier. The present chapter highlights the scope and implications of AI in childhood and adolescent disorders, with a specific highlight on diagnosis at early stages, cognitive training for attention-deficit hyperactive disorder, risk assessment of psychosis, and, most importantly, suicide risk. The chapter also highlights the ethical issues and challenges of using Ai in childhood and adolescent mental health care.

Keywords Childhood disorders · Adolescent mental health · Autism · AI-based tools

It may sound distressing and even surprising to some, but children and adolescents can have major mental health issues. Apart from disorders like Autism, Attention-Deficit Hyperactive Disorder, learning disability, intellectual disability which are diagnosed in childhood itself; children and adolescents can have major mental illnesses like adults. The Centre for Disease Control and Prevention (CDC) reports that approximately 1 in 5 children have a mental, emotional, or behavioural disorder, but fewer than 20% receive care from a mental health specialist. In India, the mental health status of adolescents—defined as individuals aged 10–19—is a significant concern. The National Mental Health Survey of India (2015–2016) reported a prevalence of psychiatric disorders among adolescents aged 13–17 at 7.3%, whereas, in the United States, this figure stands at 27.9%. This problem is exacerbated by stigma, lack of awareness, and a significant treatment gap of 95% for common mental disorders, which is even higher than the treatment gap for severe disorders (76%).

S. Halder et al., *Navigating AI in Mental Health Care*,
https://doi.org/10.1007/978-981-96-9744-1_8

On top, an early onset of major mental illness is also an indication of poorer outcome, because of inherent biological and genetic predisposition. Thus, it becomes important to identify children and adolescents at risk as early as possible.

As engagement is a key predictor of intervention effectiveness, and child and adolescent population groups are usually technology users comfortable with tech in healthcare settings, AI's value is particularly notable for this population. The anonymity provided by AI tools can help overcome the stigma surrounding mental health issues in younger populations, offering a non-judgemental resource.

AI excels in classification and prediction, showing great promise in diagnosing disorders, predicting mental health crises, and alerting healthcare practitioners. It has proven effective in predicting treatment outcomes for conditions like paediatric obsessive–compulsive disorder, attention-deficit/hyperactivity disorder, and autism across all ages. Let's see how AI is changing the landscape of processes in mental health services for the younger lot.

AI in Adolescents' Mental Health Disorder Diagnosis, Treatment, and Prognosis

Mental health spans across different stages of life, including preschool, adolescence, and adulthood and encompasses the social, psychological, and emotional well-being of an individual, influencing how they think, feel, and respond to life situations. Good mental health enables individuals to function effectively and reach their full potential. Early diagnosis of mental health issues is critical for improving patient care and understanding mental health conditions. However, diagnosing mental disorders presents unique challenges, as distinguishing between mental and physical health can be difficult. Mental health diagnoses often rely on self-reported data through targeted interrogations aimed at identifying specific patterns of behaviour and emotion, unlike other chronic illnesses that require laboratory tests. Additionally, one major challenge in treating mental health issues is the lack of mechanistic models for psychiatric disorders due to the complexity of the brain, making it difficult to clearly describe the development of a given mental illness. Recent advancements in AI, machine learning (ML), and deep learning (DL) have significantly impacted mental healthcare. AI's performance in these areas is closely linked to the availability of data, and as mental health data continues to grow, AI techniques are increasingly being applied to enhance our understanding of mental health. In recent years, DL techniques have demonstrated superior performance in diagnosis, prognosis, and treatment in the healthcare sector. AI, particularly in the form of machine learning models, is utilized to analyse medical data and derive insights that improve health outcomes and patient experiences. Mental health professionals use AI to accomplish various tasks, such as providing insights into therapy sessions, refining diagnoses, monitoring patients' conditions, and adjusting treatments as necessary.

AI for Mental Disorder Diagnosis: AI has shown significant potential in diagnosing medical disorders, including mental health conditions. Techniques, like machine learning, including the Boltzmann machine, support vector machine (SVM), and K-Nearest Neighbor (kNN), have been successfully applied to detect and diagnose diseases. Machine learning and computer vision, subsets of AI, are particularly effective due to their capabilities in imaging, segmentation, and prediction. These approaches are successful because of their emphasis on the generalizability of models to new data. For example, a deep neural network model was proposed by Khan et al. to analyse genome sequencing data in the diagnosis of schizophrenia, which is characterized by hallucinations or delusions. AI is also widely applied in diagnosing other mental health conditions. It can predict the diagnosis of new patients based on the training dataset from previous cases. Moreover, AI can differentiate between diagnoses of diseases with similar symptoms but different treatment methods. For instance, AI has been used to distinguish between bipolar and unipolar depression using brain imaging features and to differentiate types of dementia using structural MRI scans. Data-driven AI methods that incorporate demographic features, neurocognitive profiles, and biomarkers can help identify novel disease subtypes. Additionally, AI methodologies can detect patterns in data collected over long periods, which is crucial for validating diagnoses based on the evolution of psychiatric conditions. For example, Sen et al. have utilized a generative network called an autoencoder to work with fMRI and sMRI data for diagnosing ADHD, improving classification accuracy rates up to 67%.

AI in Child Development Monitoring: The use of AI in child development monitoring holds significant potential, particularly in addressing the challenges associated with early detection of developmental delays. Delayed identification of congenital or acquired diseases can exacerbate developmental issues, making timely intervention crucial. Despite the importance of regular developmental assessments across various age groups, resource constraints often limit their frequency, leading to many children with developmental delays remaining undiagnosed. This issue is further complicated by inconsistent use of standardized screening tools and significant delays between parents' initial concerns and medical consultations, particularly in low and middle-income countries where access to developmental assessments is limited. AI technologies offer a promising solution for overcoming these challenges by providing an accessible and scalable approach to monitoring child development. As healthcare becomes increasingly digitalized, AI has the potential to streamline the screening process, enhance early detection, and reduce the burden on healthcare resources. However, there is a risk that the digital divide could widen the gap between developed and underdeveloped countries, making global collaboration essential to ensure equitable access to these technologies.

Current evidence of AI use in paediatrics is limited, with most research focusing on subspecialties such as neonatology, mental health, and neurology. Autism spectrum disorder (ASD) detection is a primary area of interest, with several studies demonstrating high accuracy and specificity in diagnosing ASD. Nonetheless, there is a consensus that real-world clinical and large-scale evaluations of AI applications are lacking. Although AI has shown promise in areas like autism screening, speech analysis, sepsis prediction, and preterm care, its application in broader child development monitoring remains underexplored. One of the main challenges in implementing AI for child development monitoring is the wide range of what is considered "normal" development. The physiological variations in child development make it difficult to define pathological development without longitudinal data and expert input. Additionally, the acceptance of AI by all stakeholders is crucial for its success. While parents view digital tools as useful resources, they often question their reliability and prefer consulting with physicians. Similarly, healthcare professionals express mixed opinions about AI due to a lack of practical experience and knowledge. Integrating the expertise and insights of medical staff into AI applications is vital, particularly in the paediatric sector, to ensure the technology's effective and widespread adoption.

Early diagnosis is crucial for better outcomes, as timely interventions during critical developmental periods can significantly improve skills in communication, behaviour, and cognition. Traditional diagnostic tools like the Modified Checklist for Autism in Toddlers (M-CHAT), Autism Diagnostic Observation Schedule (ADOS) or the Childhood Autism Rating Scale (CARS) have long been effective, but advancements in AI have opened new possibilities. By analysing indicators such as speech quality, facial expressions, and motor patterns, AI tools can enable earlier and more accurate diagnosis. Detecting autism in early childhood is essential because the brain exhibits high neuroplasticity during this period. Interventions during the early years can significantly enhance a child's abilities and reduce the intensity of autism symptoms over time. However, delayed diagnosis often results from limited access to trained professionals and subjective assessment methods. Traditional tools like questionnaires and observation-based methods, while effective, may miss subtle early indicators. AI can address these gaps by identifying patterns invisible to the human eye, offering a more objective and timely approach. Interventions during the early years can significantly enhance a child's abilities and reduce the intensity of autism symptoms over time.

Let us see how AI helped in diagnosis and management of a 10-year-old boy, brought to a clinic by his parents due to concerns about delayed speech, difficulty in maintaining eye contact, and repetitive motor behaviours like hand-flapping. The family reported that these symptoms had been present since he was 2 years old but were not diagnosed due to limited awareness. AI tools leveraged advanced technologies like machine learning (ML), natural language processing (NLP), and computer vision to analyse large datasets and detect subtle patterns indicative of ASD in the boy. AI also evaluated speech quality, including pitch, rhythm, and tone of the child and variations in these parameters, such as monotonic intonation or delayed speech, are potential indicators of autism. AI software further analysed recordings of the child's speech, identifying flat intonation and irregular rhythm. AI-based models analyse video footage to detect atypical gaze patterns, reduced emotional responsiveness, or irregular facial expressions. These tools can objectively evaluate the child's engagement and social cues. Using video footage, the AI system detected reduced eye contact and atypical facial expressions during interactions. Wearable devices equipped with sensors can track repetitive behaviours and irregular motor

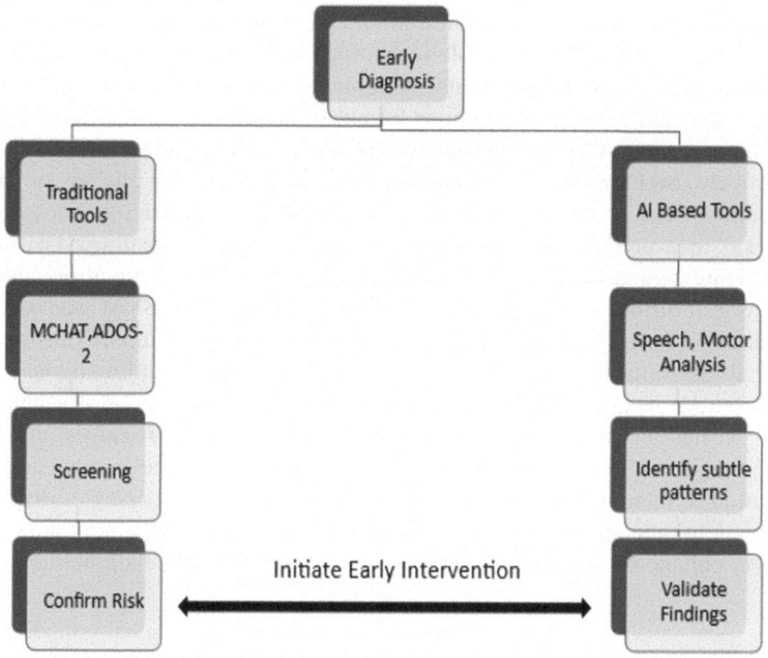

Fig. 8.1 AI implications in autism

patterns. These patterns, such as hand flapping or unusual gait, are often early signs of autism. Motion sensors tracked repetitive movements, confirming behavioural observations. The AI-assisted evaluation validated the traditional diagnosis and highlighted patterns that traditional methods might have missed earlier. This demonstrates the potential of AI in reducing diagnostic delays and refining assessments (Fig. 8.1).

AI in autism diagnosis offers several key advantages, including enhanced objectivity by minimizing variability in assessments and providing consistent, unbiased results. It enables early detection of subtle signs of autism, allowing for timely interventions that can significantly improve outcomes. Additionally, AI tools increase accessibility by being deployable in non-clinical settings like homes and schools, broadening the reach of diagnostic services. Moreover, AI systems facilitate real-time monitoring of developmental progress, enabling ongoing adjustments to intervention strategies, and supporting more personalized care. Together, these benefits contribute to a more efficient, effective, and inclusive approach to autism diagnosis and intervention.

Despite its advantages, AI faces challenges, including data diversity, privacy concerns, and ensuring reliability. AI models trained on limited datasets may fail to generalize across populations. Privacy issues arise from using sensitive data like video recordings, requiring strict compliance with regulations. Additionally, AI tools should complement, not replace, human expertise, emphasizing the clinician's role in interpreting findings. Future research should focus on developing culturally inclusive AI models, integrating wearable technology, and enhancing user-friendliness. Collaborations between technologists, clinicians, and caregivers will be essential to create practical and ethical AI solutions for autism diagnosis.

AI for treatment of Mental Disorders in Children and Adolescents: AI can also be effectively used to assess treatment responses and predict the efficacy of various drug combinations, aiding in the development of precision medicine. For example, Chang et al. measured the effectiveness of methylphenidate for treating ADHD using neuroimaging biomarkers, developing a multivariate pattern recognition approach that measured differences in volumetric information in sMRI. SVM was used as a classifier to perform binary classification between different volumetric measures.

Li et al. used machine learning models to classify normal and malignant sMRI samples based on grey matter volumetric (GMV) correlates in adolescents with ADHD. AI has the potential to revolutionize the diagnosis, prognosis, and treatment of mental health disorders, particularly in adolescents. By leveraging advanced AI techniques, mental health professionals can improve the accuracy of diagnoses, predict patient outcomes more effectively, and tailor treatments to individual needs, ultimately enhancing patient care and outcomes in the mental health field.

Application of AI in Intervention Training for ADHD

Traditional intervention trainings for ADHD have included pharmacological approaches, behaviour therapy, and cognitive training programmes utilizing paper–pencil or computerized methods. However, recent advancements in AI have introduced more precise and predictive tools for attention training, marking a significant leap in ADHD management. AI-based attention training tools are more precise and predictive than traditional methods because they leverage real-time data and advanced algorithms to tailor interventions to the individual's specific needs. Unlike standardized exercises that apply a one-size-fits-all approach, AI dynamically adapts the difficulty and nature of tasks based on moment-to-moment performance, ensuring personalized targeting of attention deficits. Additionally, these tools analyse historical data to predict future challenges, enabling proactive adjustments and minimizing inefficiencies (Fig. 8.2).

Conventional methods of attention training for ADHD primarily involve repetitive exercises aimed at improving sustained attention, selective attention, and working memory. These exercises are often limited because:

1. Standardized exercises may become monotonous and fail to engage the child.
2. Individual differences are not adequately addressed.
3. Skills developed during training often fail to transfer to real-life scenarios.

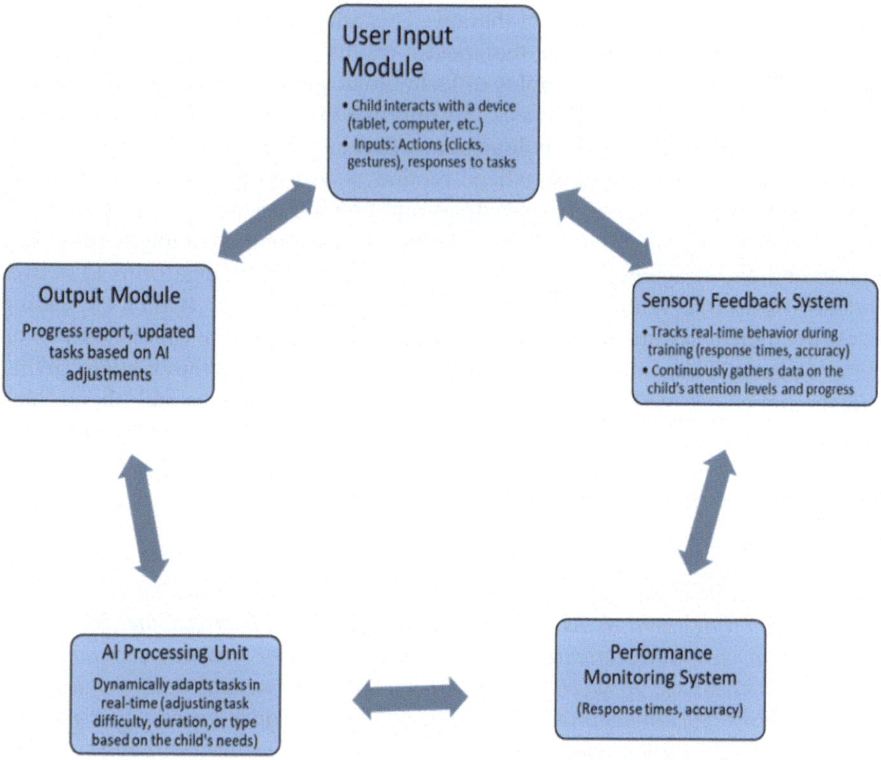

Fig. 8.2 AI augmentation in attention training for children

Advancements with AI-Based Tools

AI-based attention training tools leverage machine learning algorithms and real-time data analysis to create adaptive and engaging interventions. AI-based tasks can be adjusted in daily life to match the individual's performance and learning pace and AI can also pinpoint specific attention deficits and tailor training programmes accordingly. To improve the engagement in intervention, Gamified interfaces and immersive environments, such as virtual reality (VR), ensure to enhance user motivation. AI tools use past performance data to predict future challenges, allowing proactive adjustments which will be benefited for continuous monitoring by the therapists and caregivers. AI has great potential to improve therapy efficacy and personalization in the management of ADHD. By using AI, medical professionals can forecast how each patient will react to drugs and treatments, allowing for individualized treatment programmes based on each patient's particular traits. To find the best drug and dosage, for example, AI systems can examine genetic profiles, medical histories, and past treatment results, minimising side effects and enhancing adherence. Through wearable technology and smartphone apps, AI-powered solutions also make it possible to continuously monitor the course of therapy. This allows for real-time feedback and prompt adjustments to maximize therapeutic results. Virtual assistants and smartphone applications are two examples of technologies that help people with ADHD manage their illness on a daily basis. To improve executive functioning and self-management abilities, these technologies can offer real-time coaching, help with task organization, and send out personalized reminders. An AI-powered virtual coach, for instance, might examine daily routines and provide customized suggestions to enhance time management, lessen distractions, and sustain motivation by providing support and encouragement. AI makes it easier for interactive platforms to deliver evidence-based interventions like cognitive-behavioural therapy (CBT), expanding access to efficient treatments for people who face obstacles to conventional in-person therapy. ChatGPT can improve results by creating customized therapy content, giving patients immediate feedback, and facilitating engaging dialogues with them. Such AI-based virtual assistants are a useful complement to ADHD care because they provide scalable and easily accessible ways to provide individualized support and therapy, particularly in settings with limited resources.

Case Study

A 9-year-old child complained of poor concentration, restlessness, academic deterioration and diagnosed as ADHD. Assessment exhibited average intelligence but difficulties in sustaining attention in academic tasks. For this boy psychological intervention consisted of weekly therapist-guided sessions and daily home practice using tasks like connecting dots, number and letter cancellation, letter-number sequencing, and position coding. Parents were actively involved through psychoeducation and counselling to monitor progress. Post-intervention results indicated significant improvements in inattention, hyperactivity/impulsivity, and oppositional defiance behaviour. The program's structured and incremental design helped children enhance sustained, selective, and divided attention, while parental involvement and homework assignments reinforced learning. This intervention demonstrated that simple, structured tasks could partially improve ADHD symptoms and academic performance.

Despite undergoing traditional paper–pencil training and behavioural interventions, progress was minimal, particularly in transferring skills to home settings. He was introduced to an AI-based attention training programme using a VR platform. The programme involved completing a series of gamified attention tasks within a simulated room. Real-time feedback and adjustments were provided based on his performance. He was more motivated to participate in the training sessions due to the interactive nature of the tasks and AI identified specific challenges in selective attention and designed targeted exercises to address them through constant modifications. He also demonstrated significant improvement in academic performance, including better focus during lessons and reduced impulsivity. Thus, AI-based attention training can amplify the gains of conventional paper–pencil-based interventions (Table 8.1, Fig. 8.3).

AI-based attention training tools represent a promising future for ADHD management. By offering greater precision, adaptability, and predictability, these tools

Table 8.1 Traditional vs. AI-based attention training

Aspect	Paper–pencil	AI-driven tools
Adaptability	Fixed Tasks, one-size-fits all	Dynamic, real-time adaptation
Engagement	Low, repetitive exercises	High, gamified experiences
Precision	Generalized feedback	Tailored, specific interventions
Predictability	Minimal	High, Proactive adjustments
Transferability	Limited	Significant

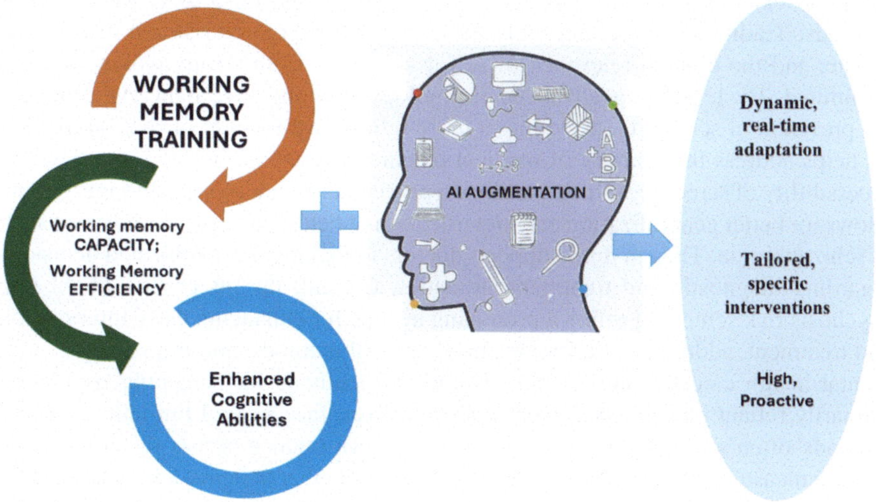

Fig. 8.3 Illustration of the AI-augmented working memory training model for ADHD

address the limitations of traditional methods. The above case exemplifies the transformative potential of such innovations, enabling children with ADHD to achieve better outcomes both academically and socially.

AI for Adolescent Psychosis Risk Screening

There is broad consensus that improving the early identification of individuals at risk for psychosis through effective screening is crucial for promoting early intervention. Traditional screening methods for psychosis, which primarily rely on various scales, often face challenges in accurately and timely identifying adolescents who are at risk. These methods can be cumbersome and may not always capture the nuanced indicators of psychosis risk in a timely manner. Recent advancements in AI have dramatically transformed many fields, including psychiatric research and practice. The explosive development of new algorithms, coupled with high-performance parallel computing, large-capacity storage, and diverse technological inputs like video, text, and sound, has accelerated the growth of AI. This rapid advancement has fostered significant improvements in how mental health conditions are treated and researched. One of the most notable benefits of AI in adolescent psychosis risk screening is its ability to enhance the speed and timeliness of identifying individuals who are either currently affected or at potential risk for psychosis. This improvement in screening efficiency facilitates early intervention and treatment, allowing for the timely correction of risky behaviours and the prevention of symptom exacerbation. AI also boosts the accuracy and objectivity of screening methods. Traditional screening tools for adolescent psychosis risk are often inadequate, and the clinical relevance of self-assessment results from adolescents can be limited. By leveraging advanced technology and objective data, AI enhances the precision of screening, providing a more reliable assessment of risk. Moreover, AI helps address the scarcity of medical resources by increasing the coverage and accessibility of screenings. Its capability to process and analyse vast amounts of data allows for better generalization and identification of heterogeneity in conditions such as schizophrenia. This, in turn, supports doctors in making more informed decisions regarding diagnostic and treatment strategies. Overall, the integration of AI into psychosis risk screening offers a promising avenue for enhancing early intervention and treatment, addressing limitations in traditional methods, and improving overall mental health care for adolescents. Traditional methods for screening psychosis, primarily reliant on self-assessment questionnaires, face several limitations. These methods often suffer from inconsistencies in performance across different tools, varying measurement criteria—including content, number of items, and thresholds—and a lack of dynamic, longitudinal tracking data. Additionally, self-assessment scales depend on individuals' self-perceptions and recollections, which can be unreliable. For instance, patients with depression might exhibit recall bias, and symptoms can fluctuate significantly over time or even throughout the day, complicating accurate and timely symptom assessment. AI has emerged as a promising solution to address these limitations. AI technologies, particularly machine learning algorithms, have evolved significantly, improving their applicability in psychosis risk screening. Traditional algorithms such as decision trees, naive Bayes, random forests, support vector machines, and K-nearest neighbours have been widely used, with support vector machines proving particularly common. More recent advancements include deep learning algorithms like convolutional neural networks, autoencoders, and deep belief networks, which offer enhanced capabilities for psychosis risk assessment. AI tools in psychosis screening often involve chatbots and large-scale social media data analysis.

Chatbot: Chatbots, which facilitate human–computer interactions through natural language processing, have advanced considerably. Initially driven by static databases and rule-based responses, modern chatbots now leverage real-time learning and evolutionary algorithms to simulate natural language communication more effectively. Examples include Tess, HealthBuddy, and Woebot. Woebot, for instance, engages users through daily conversations and mood tracking, helping to manage anxiety and depression. A study comparing Woebot with an e-book on depression found that users interacting with Woebot experienced a significant reduction in depression compared to those using the e-book, although further validation is needed. Chatbots offer several advantages, such as increasing accessibility for those previously unable to access screenings and reducing stigma associated with mental health. However, they also have limitations, including potential conflicts of interest due to commercial sponsorships, a lack of genuine emotional awareness, and issues related to privacy and ethics.

Large-scale Social Media Data Analysis: Large-scale social media data analysis represents another innovative approach to psychosis risk screening. As social media usage grows, platforms like Facebook and Twitter provide rich sources of data for identifying and predicting psychosis. AI tools that analyse textual information, emojis, user logs, and pictures can leverage natural language processing and sentiment analysis to detect mental health issues. Studies have shown that AI systems analysing social media data can accurately predict depression and other conditions. For instance, machine learning models applied to social media posts have achieved high classification accuracy for depression and other mental health conditions. Additionally, data from wearable devices and smartphone sensors can provide valuable insights into daily activities, sleep patterns, and social interactions, further enhancing predictive capabilities. The integration of AI into psychosis risk screening holds great promise for improving early identification and intervention. The continuous development of AI technologies, including chatbots and social media analysis tools, offers new opportunities for enhancing mental health care. However, it is crucial to address the limitations and challenges associated with these technologies to ensure their effective and ethical use in detecting and managing psychosis risk among adolescents.

AI to Identify Risk Factors for Suicide in Children and Adolescents

Suicide is recognized by the World Health Organization (WHO) as a critical public health issue, particularly given its significant impact across all age groups. However, this issue is especially crucial during developmental stages, as the transition from adolescence to early adulthood sees a sharp increase in suicide rates. The onset of suicidal thoughts and behaviours often occurs before the age of 25, making early identification and intervention vital. Adolescence, in particular, is a period of heightened vulnerability, with suicidal ideation and attempted suicide representing the second leading cause of death among youth aged 10–19. Despite the severity of this issue, there is still no consensus on specific terminology in the literature on suicide. Suicidal behaviours and thoughts (SBTs) encompass a continuum of symptoms that vary in severity but share common risk factors. While SBTs are closely related, they differ in terms of prevalence, intent, and lethality. Suicidal ideation is a significant risk factor for subsequent suicidal behaviour, with the likelihood of attempting suicide by age 30 being 12 times higher for individuals with a history of suicidal ideation. Importantly, suicide prevention is possible across all age groups. Given the multifactorial nature of suicide, prevention strategies must involve coordinated efforts across healthcare, education, politics, and mass media.

The WHO's Mental Health Action Plan 2013–2030 underscores the importance of reducing suicide rates globally, aiming for a one-third reduction by 2030. A critical aspect of this plan is the early detection of predictors of suicidal behaviour, which can aid in identifying at-risk individuals, planning prevention strategies, and implementing targeted therapeutic interventions. AI techniques have proven effective in identifying suicidal behaviours among psychiatrically hospitalized adolescents. A major challenge in suicidology is distinguishing between suicidal ideation and the progression to attempted or failed suicide. Self-injurious behaviours that are not intended to result in death, such as nonsuicidal self-injury (often used to regulate negative emotional states), must be differentiated from suicidal acts. Furthermore, clinical practice often distinguishes between attempted suicides—where the outcome is non-fatal due to low lethality methods or premature interruption by the individual—and failed suicides, where a fatal outcome is avoided due to external intervention, despite high lethality methods and confirmed suicidal intent.

AI for Mental Disorder Prognosis: AI's strong predictive power and generalization abilities make it a valuable tool for the prognosis of mental disorders. AI techniques can analyse longitudinal data from psychiatric patients, including neuroimaging, genetic and electronic health records to provide accurate prognoses. For instance, Koutsouleris et al. collected MRI and genotyping data from psychiatric patients with high-risk syndromes and recent-onset depression to predict psychosis using SVM techniques. SVM was used to classify patients into high-risk, recent-onset, and normal control categories based on learned features from multimodal data. Electroencephalogram (EEG) signals have been used as valuable brain data for mental disorder prognosis. Zhdanov et al. used resting-state EEG signals to predict the effectiveness of specific drugs for depression, employing a radial basis function (RBF) SVM to estimate treatment effectiveness. This model achieved an accuracy of 82.4% in classifying different severities of disorders. Similarly, studies by Geng and Xu, as well as Nieuwenhuis et al., analysed neuroimaging data using DL techniques like autoencoders and CNN to perform prognosis studies on patients with depression and schizophrenia. Smucny et al. also investigated the clinical improvement of psychosis patients using fMRI data, comparing the performance of various ML and DL models. They found multilayer neural networks performed well with fMRI data, achieving a prognosis accuracy of 70%.

Issues and Challenges

While AI holds great promise for improving accessibility, efficiency, and precision in mental health interventions, its application in such a sensitive and vulnerable population must be approached with caution. The use of AI in mental health care, particularly with children and adolescents, presents a range of ethical and practical concerns.

One of the foremost concerns is data security and privacy. The collection and processing of sensitive mental health data, especially from minors, require robust safeguards to prevent unauthorized access, misuse, or breaches. Children and adolescents are particularly vulnerable to the consequences of data breaches, which could result in stigmatization, bullying, or even future discrimination.

The challenge lies in ensuring that AI systems are not only secure but also transparent about how data is collected, stored, and used. It's crucial to establish clear guidelines and regulations that protect young users' privacy while enabling the potential benefits of AI in mental health care.

Informed consent is another critical issue, especially when dealing with minors who may not fully understand the implications of their data being used by AI tools. Obtaining informed consent from children and adolescents requires careful consideration of their developmental stage and cognitive abilities. The process must involve clear, age-appropriate explanations of how the AI functions, what data it collects, and the potential risks involved. Additionally, parental or guardian consent should be required, ensuring that all parties involved are fully informed and agreeable to the AI's use.

AI systems are only as good as the data they are trained on, and there is a significant risk of bias in these systems. If the data used to train AI models is not representative of diverse populations, the AI may produce biased outcomes, which can perpetuate existing disparities in mental health care. For instance, AI might underdiagnose or misdiagnose conditions in certain racial or ethnic groups due to a lack of diverse data. This is particularly concerning in a population as diverse as children and adolescents, where developmental, cultural, and social factors significantly influence mental health. It is essential to ensure that AI systems are trained on diverse datasets and are regularly audited for bias to provide fair and equitable care.

Another concern is the lack of empathy and contextual understanding that AI systems inherently possess. Mental health care often relies on the nuanced understanding and empathy of a human therapist, who can provide emotional support and tailor interventions based on the unique context of each patient. AI, however, operates on algorithms and data, lacking the ability to understand the emotional depth or the specific life circumstances of a child or adolescent. This limitation raises questions about the appropriateness of using AI in therapeutic settings where human connection and empathy are critical.

The problem of AI "Hallucination": AI chatbots, which are increasingly being used in mental health care, have been known to "hallucinate", meaning they can generate false or misleading information with unwarranted confidence. This is particularly dangerous in mental health applications, where incorrect or harmful advice could exacerbate a young person's condition. The possibility of an AI chatbot providing inaccurate or harmful guidance underscores the importance of human oversight and the need for clear protocols to manage and mitigate these risks.

AI offers exciting possibilities for enhancing mental health care for children and adolescents, its implementation must be approached with caution. Addressing concerns around data security, privacy, informed consent, bias, empathy, and AI hallucination is essential to ensure that these technologies are safe, ethical, and effective in supporting the mental health of young people. The role of AI should be to complement, not replace, human therapists, ensuring that the unique needs of each child or adolescent are met with the care and sensitivity they deserve.

Looking to the future, technological advancements in AI for paediatric mental health are expected to be both dramatic and rapid. However, the major obstacle is not the technology itself but the governance and regulation of these tools. Currently, there is a lack of consensus on standards for AI in health care, and the field remains largely unregulated in the United.States. This creates a significant challenge in ensuring that AI applications are safe, effective, and ethical. The need for a regulatory body analogous to the U.S. Food and Drug Administration (FDA) for AI in health care is becoming increasingly apparent. Such an organization could establish and enforce standards, oversee the development and deployment of AI tools, and ensure that these technologies meet rigorous safety and efficacy criteria before they are widely used. While the concerns surrounding AI in paediatric mental health are valid, they should not necessarily lead to a rejection of AI technologies. Instead, these concerns highlight the need for thoughtful regulation and the development of professional standards. Just as we address issues like bias and privacy breaches in human therapists, similar vigilance is required for AI tools. The current paediatric mental health crisis, marked by widespread need and limited resources, underscores the importance of integrating AI into mental health care. AI has the potential to augment human efforts, providing support where it is most needed and extending the reach of mental health services. However, this potential can only be fully realized if we address the associated risks through comprehensive regulation and continuous oversight. By doing so, we can harness the benefits of AI while minimizing its risks, ultimately improving outcomes for children and adolescents in need of mental health support.

Conclusion

The application of AI in managing childhood and adolescent disorders has brought a new dimension to understanding and treating mental health challenges in young individuals. AI offers the potential to revolutionize the way mental health care is delivered by focusing on precision, accessibility, and effectiveness. It provides unique tools to personalize treatments, monitor progress, and optimize outcomes, making it a powerful ally in addressing complex mental health issues. By analysing factors such as genetic profiles, clinical histories, and previous outcomes, AI algorithms can help healthcare professionals determine the most effective therapies and medications for a specific individual. This minimizes trial-and-error methods, reduces adverse effects, and improves treatment adherence, particularly in disorders like ADHD and depression. AI-powered tools can also monitor behavioural patterns through wearable devices and smartphone applications, offering real-time feedback that enables timely intervention and adjustments to therapeutic strategies. Beyond treatment, AI enhances self-management and executive functioning in young individuals with mental health disorders. AI-driven virtual assistants and mobile applications provide personalized reminders, organize daily tasks, and offer real-time coaching to help children and adolescents stay on track with their routines. For instance, these tools can suggest strategies to improve focus, manage time efficiently, and overcome distractions, fostering better coping mechanisms in daily life. This level of support not only empowers young individuals but also reduces the burden on caregivers and families.

Chapter 9
AI for Dementia and Other Memory Problems

Abstract With declining age comes decline in cognitive functions and daily living with independence becomes a challenge. For some people this decline is age appropriate, but for some the decline is grave enough to be diagnosed as mild cognitive impairment or further as dementia, characterized by progressive difficulties in memory, reasoning, and communication. Dementia is a persistent loss of cognition in multiple cognitive domains severe enough to limit social or occupational function. It is quantitatively and qualitatively different from age-related cognitive decline in the elderly and is a disabling condition. In absence of a cure for dementia, the focus lies in management of dementia, where early diagnosis, and supportive care are important. In this chapter, we primarily discuss dementia and the progressive implications of AI in its diagnosis and management.

Keywords Dementia · Memory problems · Old age · AI in diagnosis

The Ticking Clock of Time

Shalini (name changed), aged 74 years, sat in the lawn of her home gazing at the fading hues of the sunset. She looked at the tall peach tree, which she and her husband had planted several years ago. It was full of bloom, and just one of the reminders of the lovely times she had with her husband in this house. She had spent almost fifty years in the house and every nook and corner of the house had a story of her husband, children and of course hers. Those moments felt like they belonged to a different lifetime. She lived alone in the house as her children worked in different cities and visited her on regular intervals and holidays. As she poured tea with her trembling hands, she was happy as her younger son had called and mentioned he was visiting with his family next week, but she was also bothered and felt helpless for being unable to recall her grandson's birthday. Her memory was not as good as before. Age, once an abstract concept, had become her daily reality. With aging came challenges she hadn't anticipated—her body, once strong, was slowing, and her mind was clouded by forgetfulness and confusion. She retired as a manager in a public

S. Halder et al., *Navigating AI in Mental Health Care*,
https://doi.org/10.1007/978-981-96-9744-1_9

bank and had a satisfactory work record. Though before retirement she was not as sharp, and there were occasions when she missed signing important documents on time. Her senior manager shared good rapport with her and advised her not to engage in important office matters before retirement, which was due shortly. Post-retirement life had been peaceful for Shalini and her husband as they toured places, visited their children and spent most of their time gardening until three years back when her husband succumbed to cardiac arrest. Both had contracted COVID-19 during the first wave and though recovered gradually, her husband was much weaker than before. Shalini too was not her usual self and gradually required more assistance in daily living. The shift from independence to dependency was humbling and even isolating. She wondered if others noticed her struggle to find words during conversations or her hesitance in navigating once-familiar paths to the supermarket for grocery or other places. She was okay with computers due to her prior work life but found the new smartphones and apps a bit tricky to handle with their constant updates, and worried for the gradual shift of everyday affairs from bill payments to availing of other services linked with mobile phones. The story of Shalini is not just hers but millions of men and women of her age around the globe who are diagnosed with dementia and struggle with activities of daily life.

As the life cycle progresses, old age emerges as an inevitable phase, often marked by profound biological, psychological, and social transitions and conditions like diabetes, cardiovascular illness, vision and hearing impairment, high blood pressure, skeletal-muscle weakness to name a few. The physical vigour of youth gradually gives way to declining energy levels, reduced mobility, and an increased susceptibility to chronic illnesses. Similarly, cognitive functions—such as memory, attention, and problem-solving—may begin to falter, signalling the subtle but impactful changes in the brain associated with aging. This phase of life also brings with it significant psychosocial challenges. Psychosocial support undertakes certain changes as children may move to different places due to marriage or work, and elderly relatives are no more. The loss of professional roles, changes in family dynamics, and diminishing social interactions can contribute to feelings of isolation, sadness, and anxiety. Yet, it is within this stage that individuals often seek to find new meaning and purpose, demonstrating resilience in the face of life's inevitable transitions. However, it is important to remain fit both physically and mentally in old age, where many people falter.

Overview of Dementia: Dementia is usually connected with a variety of neuropathologies, the most notable of which are Alzheimer's disease and cerebrovascular pathology. According to the Lancet Commission, dementia is "the greatest worldwide concern for social and health care services in the twenty-first century". It is a progressive pathological neurological condition of the brain that results in a syndrome of diminished thinking, memory, behaviour, and function. A reduced quality of life and growing difficulty doing daily tasks are associated with dementia. Due mostly to ageing populations, more than 50 million people worldwide suffer from dementia, and by 2050, that number is expected to rise to an astounding 152 million. In addition to being a substantial healthcare expense that costs over $1 trillion annually, dementia has a tremendous human cost for both patients and their families.

Dementia is not a single disease, but rather a collection of symptoms linked to underlying disorders such as vascular Alzheimer's disease, frontotemporal dementia, or Lewy body dementia. Aside from forgetfulness, people with dementia may have trouble with expressing themselves through language, impaired judgement, and fluctuations in mood and behavioural patterns, and a reduction in their ability to accomplish basic daily chores. The symptoms frequently develop with time and can significantly impair the individual's standard of life and productivity. Dementia can develop at any age. However, the possibility of dementia increases with years of age, and it is more common in persons over the age of 60. Other risk factors for dementia include genetics, elevated blood pressure, smoking, diabetes, and obesity.

Prevalence and Impact

In the United States, 5.8 million people suffer from Alzheimer's disease. The number of people with dementia worldwide is expected to triple from existing numbers to 152 million by the year 2050 as the global population gets older with a longer life span. Progression into dementia doesn't happen overnight. While many cases have been recorded in the world's richest and most aged countries, nearly 63% of people who suffer from dementia live in countries with low or middle incomes with limited availability of social protection, services, support, and care.

Improving population health has the potential to reduce the future dementia epidemic by 10–20%, according to current projections.

Dementia is amongst the most common chronic diseases that cause disability in the elderly globally. In individuals who have advanced forms of dementia, the last year of life is marked by a pattern of chronic severe disability. The Global Deterioration Scale describes advanced dementia with profound memory deficits, minimal verbal abilities, being unable to move around independently, inability to manage daily activities, and urinary and faecal incontinence.

Although elderly individuals can frequently manage well, and continue to be somewhat independent, cognitive impairment rapidly impairs a person's capacity to perform difficult yet necessary everyday duties. Additionally, it will become more difficult for those suffering from dementia to meet their basic personal care demands. The requirement for a caregiver's assistance frequently begins early in the dementia process, gets worse as the condition worsens over time, and lasts until death. Numerous studies attest to the magnitude of the stress that carers endure at three levels: practically (the hours spent providing care take away from other activities, especially socializing and leisure), psychologically (emotional strain, which contributes to an elevated incidence of anxiety and depressive symptoms), and economically (increased costs, combined with giving up or reducing work to care). Multiple health issues are common in older adults, such as long-term physical illnesses that coexist with psychological or cognitive impairments. These conditions can have complicated interactions that result in disability and care needs. However, research from low- and middle-income countries as well as high-income nations agrees that dementia and cognitive impairment account for the majority of care demands among older adults, far more so than other forms of impairment and other chronic illnesses.

Can Dementia Be Prevented? Changes in exposure to hypothesized developmental, lifestyle, and cardiovascular risk factors for dementia may theoretically lead to a decrease in the age-specific probability of dementia, at least in high-income nations. The 2014 World Alzheimer Report examined the evidence basis for modifiable risk factors for dementia with an emphasis on dementia risk reduction. The most compelling evidence for potential causal links to dementia was found for early life low education, midlife hypertension, and lifelong diabetes and smoking. An 8.3% decrease in dementia prevalence through 2050 would result from a 10% reduction in these and other major risk exposures, according to a recent modelling exercise. A 15% decrease in dementia prevalence is expected in response to a twenty per cent decrease in exposure prevalence.

Population-based research is necessary to monitor the effectiveness of measures aimed at reducing dementia risk factors, such as increased education. These initiatives should prioritise adapting care arrangements and improving access to and availability of social care and healthcare services. It is desired to develop cost-effective clinical and social care packages for dementia patients and carers, including evidence-based preventative interventions. Investing in research and cost-effective care can help manage future societal costs.

Understanding Dementia and Memory Problems

As there is a certain level of decline in cognitive functions with age, it is important to differentiate age-related cognitive decline from dementia. Elderly people with age-appropriate cognitive decline are generally able to continue with their daily activities. The vocabulary and verbal skills remain largely unchanged, but they might struggle to find a particular word during conversation. Long-term memory, general knowledge and the ability to use skills and knowledge mostly remains unaffected; but forming new memories, working memory (e.g. recalling an address) is particularly affected. They are largely able to focus on a single task but have increased difficulty with multitasking or switching attention.

In contrast, patients with dementia would have marked difficulty in executing simple daily tasks. Typical presentation reported by family members include 'not being able to follow the sequence of tasks of daily living.' Memory impairments are prominent and marked even for recent events and long term. They may struggle with rational decision-making, communication, and comprehension, leading to unintentional repetition of phrases and enquiries during talks. Changes in personality patterns like increased rigidity and irritability may develop. They have problems navigating familiar environments, and difficulty performing everyday tasks are common challenges.

Symptoms Presentations

A progressive neurological disease, dementia impairs behaviour, memory, cognition, and the capacity to carry out daily tasks. Early (mild), middle (moderate), and late (severe) stages are the three primary stages that it usually progresses through; each having its unique symptoms and functional limitations. Effective recognition, diagnosis, and management of dementia depend on an understanding of the clinical manifestations at each stage.

A. Early-Stage Dementia: Early-stage dementia symptoms are frequently mild and could be confused with stress or ageing. In most cases, the first obvious symptom is memory loss. Short-term memory problems, such as remembering recent occurrences, appointments, or discussions, are common in people with early-stage dementia. They typically have no trouble recalling old memories and routines, but they have trouble remembering new material. For instance, someone might regularly lose things like glasses or keys, or they might neglect to finish a task they just started. Another sign of mild dementia is difficulty speaking. During talks, people may struggle to find the correct words, which could result in ambiguous explanations or pauses as they look for keywords. This can also show up in written communication, when words are frequently misused, or sentence structures become simpler. The majority of people at this stage, however, still have enough awareness to identify these mistakes, which can cause annoyance, shame, and social disengagement. Early dementia is also frequently accompanied by impaired judgement and decision-making. People may process knowledge or make decisions more slowly, particularly in complex situations that call for several stages or the recall of previous acts. Additionally, they could display modest personality changes, such being more apathetic or worried, which could be a response to their cognitive deterioration. Although they may require reminders or help with things like monetary management or medications, people in this phase typically maintain their independence despite these symptoms.
B. Mid-Stage Dementia: More severe cognitive and functional impairments that affect day-to-day functioning are indicative of the intermediate stage of dementia. As memory loss worsens, people find it harder to recall their past, familiar locations, and the names of people they know. They may struggle to remember important historical events in addition to recent ones, which can affect their sense of self and cause problems in their relationships with friends and family. In moderate dementia, language impairments become increasingly noticeable. People regularly lose track of talks, forget things they know, or use

the wrong phrases, which makes their speech erratic or difficult to understand. As language processing skills deteriorate, reading and writing challenges frequently accompany this. Individuals in this phase may also show signs of uncertainty regarding location and time. For instance, they could not be aware of the time of day, the season, or where they are, which might make them more anxious and cause them to ask the same questions over and over again concerning these fundamentals. In middle-stage dementia, anger, irritability, and restlessness are among the behavioural and psychological symptoms that frequently manifest. Some people suffer from illusions, thinking that those they love are strangers or that people are taking from them. Although less frequent, hallucinations can still happen and frequently involve disturbing visuals or noises for the person experiencing them. Both the person suffering from dementia and their carers may find these behavioural and perceptual changes upsetting because they can cause paranoia or mistrust in familiar situations. More severe deficits in day-to-day functioning are another symptom of middle-stage dementia. As fine motor skills along with coordination gradually deteriorate, seemingly regular tasks like dressing, bathing, and meal preparation become more difficult. People frequently require assistance with following instructions, keeping personal hygiene, and selecting appropriate attire. They run a higher risk of falling if their sense of balance and spatial awareness diminish. To protect their safety and well-being, the majority of people now need monitoring or help with everyday tasks.

C. Late-Stage Dementia: Significant cognitive deterioration and complete reliance on others for care are hallmarks of late-stage dementia. Significant memory loss occurs; people frequently become unaware of their environment, themselves, and those around them, especially close relatives. The ability to communicate is severely limited, and communication is either reduced to single words or short sentences, if it exists at all. Certain people may stop speaking altogether and simply react to emotional cues or sounds they know. Physical abilities are severely compromised in severe dementia, frequently making it unable to walk, sit unassisted, or regulate fundamental body processes. Simple tasks like turning in bed or handling utensils require assistance due to a loss of fine and gross motor abilities. Malnutrition, dehydration, and an increased risk of aspiration pneumonia can result from the usual swallowing difficulties that occur at this stage. People with severe dementia frequently require assistance with all facets of nutrition, hydration, and personal care because of these problems. At this point, behavioural symptoms could include disengagement, apathy, and unresponsiveness. Nonetheless, some people display agitation, repetitive actions, or distressing cries, which may be brought on by discomfort in the body or a failure to express their demands. Although mood symptoms like anxiety or despair might exist, they are hard to diagnose because of the restricted ability to communicate. Additionally, some people respond significantly to touch, loud noises, or bright lights because to their enhanced sensitivity to sensory inputs. As the emphasis moves from attempting to maintain cognitive function to optimising comfort and quality of life, palliative and supportive care are frequently given priority during this phase. It becomes crucial to manage pain and avoid consequences like infections and pressure sores. The severe physical, emotional, and logistical demands of end-stage dementia can be difficult for carers to handle and frequently call for specialized treatment, such as hospice or 24-h care.

Diagnosing Dementia

To diagnose dementia, a history of cognitive decline and impairment in daily activities, supported by an extended mental status examination by an expert, is required, who looks for difficulties in memory, speech, concentration, visuospatial cognition including perception of space, executive functioning, and state of mind. Brief memory impairment screening questionnaires can assist to commence and organize cognitive assessments. Screening for mental health should examine cognitive and affective states using standardized instruments like the Mini-Mental State Examination (MMSE), which is widely available, user-friendly, and has norms modified for educational status and age. In addition, comprehensive testing can help identify the extent and pattern associated with cognitive impairment, aiding in differential diagnosis. CT or MRI scans of the brain can detect structural lesions such as infarction, neoplasms, extracerebral fluid accumulation, and hydrocephalus that may cause dementia. If the patient has motor impairment, such as inflexibility, reflexive asymmetry, or aberrant reactions, MRI may be necessary to detect strokes or ischaemic alterations not seen by CT. While imaging produces modest yields similar to laboratory screening, more testing is required if the preliminary screening is unreliable. Neuropsychological testing provides more precise information on deficiencies than screening assessments, aiding in differential diagnosis. However, the existing methods comes with their own limitations, paper–pencil-based cognitive assessments, could be laborious and unresponsive to the preclinical stage. On the other hand, specialized brain imaging and body fluid markers do help in diagnosis, but their cost and intrusiveness prevent widespread usage.

To identify the presence of Alzheimer's along with additional dementias early on, we need objective and affordable biomarkers. Early patient recruitment would increase the likelihood that therapy studies would be successful, and risk factor reduction might prevent a significant number of cases.

AI in the Diagnosis of Dementia and Memory Problems

Considering the fact that a significantly high percentage of people diagnosed with mild cognitive impairment (MCI) develop dementia, early detection of MCI is important, as there are many individuals with MCI who do not convert into dementia. Thus, it is vital for researchers to look for markers that can highlight the risk of developing dementia.

Case Example
Biplab (name changed) is a 58-year-old male working in a private firm, and was presented with complaints of forgetfulness, reduced talk, and increased irritability for past 6 months.

Further history taking and clinical interview revealed significant changes in his usual behaviour like poor performance in work, missing deadlines, less participation in social activities. He was sleeping and eating less than before, which family members thought were due to his increasing age. He had been unmindful and forgetting things where he kept his things and if he had completed his daily activity tasks. Family members initially thought these as part of his growing age and did not pay much heed, as there were no signs of physical illness. Biplab consulted a general physician, who prescribed him some nutritional supplements, and mild antidepressants. However, there was not much improvement. He was gradually very less expressive and very less frequent at social gatherings. In further worsening of symptoms, he had significant difficulty identifying distant relatives or neighbours and struggled with reading and writing. Biplab was taken to a neurologist after 6–8 months of these complaints, where he was diagnosed with early phase of dementia.

Clients like Biplab with diagnosis of dementia are common while aging, though the initial consultation is more likely to be with a general physician for general medical conditions like diabetes, arthritis, kidney and bladder problems, glaucoma, lung and cardiovascular disease, and most of the time cognitive decline is missed or not part of management.

It might be common to attribute the cognitive decline and memory loss in elderly on account of age, but if they are due to MCI or early stage of dementia, this creates a significant void and delay in appropriate management of the patient and impacts outcome. Even though the existing approaches of early identification of individuals at risk of dementia or in early stage are based on sound scientific research, it often requires expert filtering of clinical data, behavioural observation, and neuropsychological evaluation cross-sectionally which appears difficult for a significant number of patients owing to infrastructural limitations.

Role of AI

AI could be highly implicated in these scenarios. In the existing non AI-based approaches, diagnosis of dementia is usually made by a specialist physician who conducts a number of clinical evaluations, such as getting a personal and informant history of cognitive impairment, a physical examination, paper–pencil-based cognitive tests, blood tests to exclude out other dementia mimics (like deficiencies in vitamin B12 levels), and MRI scans to check for localized atrophy of the brain. The entire diagnosis process depends largely on the clinician's interpretation and is costly, time-consuming, and somewhat subjective. There is a larger scope of extracting more information from a single test, reducing subjective judgement errors,

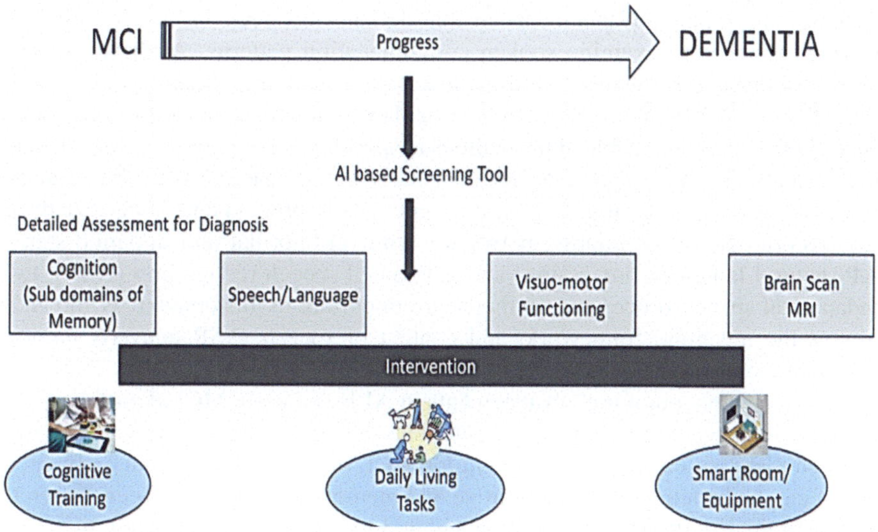

Fig. 9.1 AI implications in dementia

as well as automating the whole process of dementia screening which AI models are capable of.

As we can deduce from the following figure, the screening process needs to be augmented with AI-based models for better accuracy and confidence in screening dementia at an early stage (Fig. 9.1).

AI-based computerized cognitive assessments increase discrimination sensitivity by about 4% and specificity by about 3% when compared to traditional cognitive tests. Combining linguistic and acoustic data yields the greatest results in speech, conversation, and language exams, with an accuracy of about 94%. The accuracy of brain scan analysis using deep learning techniques is approximately 92%. The diagnosis of dementia may become more accurate and efficient with the use of machine learning (ML). Because AD is the most common cause of dementia, previous machine learning techniques have mostly concentrated on using neuroimaging data to differentiate between people with normal cognition (NC) and those with dementia and mild cognitive impairment (MCI).

In order to create an algorithm for distinguishing and, consequently, identifying cognitive impairment in patients, Kang et al. used the Seoul Neuropsychological Screening Battery, a tool often used in Korea for evaluating cognitive performance in patients with neurological illnesses. Their model shows 96.66% accuracy in detecting MCI and 79% preciseness in the three-way categorization of normal cognition, MCI, and Alzheimer's disease dementia. Similarly, Boettcher et al. and Ghoraani et al. have used gait data obtained during the dual-task assessment to investigate the detection of MCI. They showed an accuracy of MCI identification ranging from 78% to 81.52% using gradient tree enhancing machine learning models and Support Vector Machines.

One of the major advancements in this domain has been the speech classification approaches to examine spoken communication patterns. AI-driven speech processing has a great deal of promise to improve dementia diagnosis and monitoring. People with dementia frequently struggle with memory, cognition, and focus, which shows up as noticeable abnormalities in speech and language that can be identified in neuropsychological tests. By concentrating on characteristics like pauses, choices of words, and grammar, AI models are able to process and categorize these audio recordings, differentiating between cognitively normal and impaired states. NLP (natural language processing) and automated speech recognition (ASR), two fundamental speech-processing methods, are important in this context: While NLP assesses the meaning, framework, and context of speech, ASR converts phrases spoken into text for analysis.

Given recent encouraging advancements in AI-based early MCI identification, it is realistic to expect improved patient outcomes due to the ability to intervene early. Although there isn't a specific treatment for MCI, there is evidence that early intervention can be beneficial. Both cognitive and memory training have been shown to increase brain activity on neuroimaging and improve memory functioning. Improvements in AI for MCI detection have the potential to significantly impact the overall care of patients undergoing neurocognitive decline, especially in the light of the evidence of better results with earlier intervention.

How AI Applications Are Impacting Prognosis in Dementia

AI presents new opportunities for comprehending the course of dementia and enhancing outcomes for those impacted by this complicated illness owing to its capacity to evaluate enormous volumes of data, spot trends, and generate predictions. AI-based technologies hold great promise for detecting dementia symptoms early, predicting the course of the illness, customizing treatment regimens, and allocating resources in healthcare systems as efficiently as possible. Undoubtedly early cognitive decline identification is one of the most beneficial uses of AI in dementia prognosis. In the past, it has been difficult to diagnose dementia in its early stages since its symptoms are frequently mild and can mimic those of aging. In order to identify minor indicators and trends that point to early-stage dementia or even preclinical stages, AI-powered algorithms can analyse data from a range of sources, such as neurological scans, genetic profiles, and neuropsychological assessments. To find alterations in the brain's structure and function that could indicate cognitive decline, algorithms that use machine learning can be trained using datasets of cerebral magnetic resonance imaging or PET scans. As a result, patients and their families can make well-informed decisions regarding their future care and physicians can act sooner, thereby delaying the development. AI is also helpful in predicting how dementia will progress, which is crucial for personalized care and treatment planning. AI can forecast a person's dementia progression by evaluating data from longitudinal research and calculating the onset and intensity of symptoms. Algorithms, for instance, can determine variables that can affect a person's likelihood of developing Alzheimer's disease in the coming years if they now have mild cognitive impairment (MCI).

Since different people might profit from different kinds of interventions depending on their risk profiles and rates of advancement, this information is essential for personalizing care. Furthermore, AI can offer predictive knowledge into symptom patterns, including the probability of behavioural symptoms arising, enabling carers to foresee and manage potential problems in the future. AI's ability to optimize clinical decision-making and resource allocation is a noteworthy advantage in dementia prognosis.

AI systems can assist medical professionals in identifying specific treatment needs that would work best for each patient. By identifying patients who might need more intense support, AI systems may assist in managing healthcare resources better and increase the effectiveness of care delivery. Through predictive modelling, patients who are more likely to experience rapid deterioration can be identified helping in decisions about care locations, such as whether personal care homes or assisted living residences would be more suitable. Even while AI has a lot to offer in terms of dementia prognosis, there are still obstacles to overcome before these tools can be used in clinical settings. Since AI significantly depends on sizable datasets including sensitive data, it is imperative to ensure confidentiality and ethical utilization of personal health data. Furthermore, to guarantee that AI algorithms yield accurate findings across a range of demographics and clinical contexts, thorough validation is required.

AI Application in Treatment of Dementia

Research on dementia has extensively used artificial intelligence (AI). One of the most advanced machine learning techniques, deep neural networks are frequently utilized with genetic and neuroimaging data because they may identify early dementia onset and generate predictions by finding generalizable nonlinear latent patterns. AI has also been used to inform other clinical characteristics, such as aberrant changes in speech, walking, and drawing, in order to efficiently track the development of diseases and the health of the brain. AI-driven technology, such as smart sensors and robots, has been developed to manage dementia, but mostly to enhance caregiving and management. Few or no studies have been conducted to date regarding the personalization of medications in patients with dementia. However, some studies have looked into how to customize nonpharmacological interventions, such as the recommendation for physical exercise, customized interactive reminiscence sessions, etc.

AI Software's in Post-Dementia Diagnosis Support

AI-based software is becoming more and more important in helping people with dementia in receiving post-diagnosis care. It offers both direct patient aid and all-encompassing carer support. AI-powered apps can track symptoms, keep an eye on physical and mental health metrics, and alert carers or medical professionals to any notable changes in a patient's behaviour or health. For example, wearable technology with AI algorithms regularly evaluates a patient's level of activity, sleep habits, and mobility, providing carers with critical information about their daily routines and general health. Early condition diagnosis made possible by such ongoing monitoring allows for prompt therapies that can enhance quality of life and halt the progression of disease. Chatbots and virtual assistants driven by AI also offer assistance by reminding users to take their medications, schedule appointments, and do other necessary duties. By conversing with patients via natural language processing, these AI companions provide a sense of camaraderie and reinforce routines, which may help dementia sufferers feel less anxious and more independent. Additionally, by centralizing patient data to expedite care planning and interventions, AI platforms improve coordination and communication between family members, carers, and medical professionals. AI software provides a useful framework for individualized dementia care by streamlining daily administration and providing real-time health insights, ultimately improving patient outcomes and carer resilience.

AI Applications in Improving Quality of Life in Dementia Patients

Dementia impacts not only individuals but also the caregivers, often family members, who bear significant emotional and physical burdens. Advances in artificial intelligence (AI) have the potential to transform dementia care, promoting independence and reducing caregiver strain.

AI-powered wearable devices, such as smart glasses, are emerging as innovative tools to support daily living for dementia patients. These devices incorporate technologies like facial and object recognition to help users navigate their environment, recall familiar faces, and perform routine tasks with greater ease. Features such as virtual personal assistants provide reminders for medication, hydration, and meals in a familiar, emotionally comforting voice, fostering trust and connection. Additionally, caregivers benefit from complementary mobile apps that enable remote monitoring of patients' health and activities, offering real-time insights and ensuring safety. By integrating AI and Augmented Reality (AR), these tools combine practical functionality with emotional support, bridging gaps in care and enhancing quality of life for both patients and caregivers. Such innovations illustrate the promise of AI in addressing the complex challenges of dementia, paving the way for more personalized and effective solutions in geriatric mental health care (Fig. 9.2).

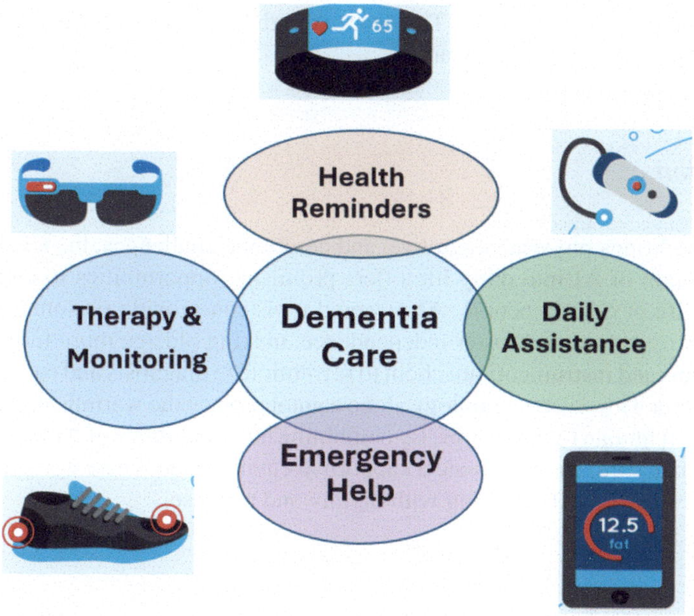

Fig. 9.2 Wearable technologies augmented with AI can enhance quality of life in dementia

Modern wearable technology comes in different forms and is getting smaller and smaller in size yet more efficient than its predecessors. The wearable technologies at present generally include smartwatches, fitness bands or trackers, virtual reality headsets, smart jewellery, web-enabled glasses and Bluetooth headsets. Not all of them have similar embedment of AI and most are individually synced with a smartphone but do provide valuable data. It may sound a far-fetched idea, but syncing multiple technologies into one to provide real-time feedback of patients is feasible and many prototypes are already available. This might be tricky or even cumbersome to make elderly people wear multiple devices for different functions at the same time; but they can be synced through cloud and provide valuable feedback both for the elderly individual as well as the caregivers.

There is credible advancement in development of social robots that are responsive machines that could provide dementia patients with company and improve their emotional or mental well-being and may not require full-time presence of caregivers. By reducing the need for constant physical presence, this type of proactive monitoring frees up the carer to concentrate on other crucial facets of care. Without being in the same room all the time, carers can deliver the finest care possible thanks to real-time updates on a patient's activities and general health. The mental strain on carers is much lessened by this kind of monitoring.

These companions can lead patients through routine activities, have thought-provoking conversations with them, or just offer comfort when they're feeling anxious. By doing this, AI improves the patient's quality of life while providing carers with much-needed breaks. This work though has scope of further refinement, fills important gaps in dementia care.

Conclusion

While aging brings physical, cognitive, and emotional challenges, the advancement and integration of AI into daily life offers promising opportunities to enhance the quality of life of elderly people. AI-powered tools can provide personalized assistance, improve safety, and foster independence, making old age more fulfilling. AI-based models and instruments are about to revolutionize diagnosis and care of elderly with dementia. However, technology alone cannot replace the warmth, empathy, and connection of human relationships. By combining the capabilities of AI with compassionate human care, we can create a supportive environment where aging is not just about surviving but truly thriving with dignity and purpose.

Part III
Upgrading Mental Health Care with AI

Chapter 10
Mitigating the Challenges for AI-Assisted Intervention in Mental Health

Abstract As the integration of AI and extensive healthcare datasets is at the cusp of revolutionizing the field of mental health care, it comes with its own challenges, apprehensions and speculations. In previous chapters, we have discussed in general about the implications of AI-based applications in different mental health conditions. In this chapter, we discuss how the intricate processes of psychodiagnostics and psychotherapy could be assisted with AI, and how to overcome the challenges in utilizing AI in mental health. This comprehensive elaboration will explore the multifaceted ways in which AI can assist in the intervention and treatment of mental health disorders, focusing on its capabilities in prediction, detection, and treatment, as well as the ethical and practical implications of these technologies. We also give an insight into the process of developing chatbots in mental health and the challenges.

Keywords Psychotherapy · Challenges · Virtual reality · Chatbot

Overview

Psychotherapy has a rich and diverse history that stretches back to ancient civilizations. Rooted in the quest for mental well-being, its evolution has been shaped by philosophical, spiritual, and scientific traditions from around the world. While modern psychotherapy is often traced to the late nineteenth century with pioneers like Sigmund Freud, its origins go much deeper, drawing on ancient practices of introspection, dialogue, and healing, the new age therapies are much more open for integrating supportive approaches and use of technology at different levels.

Ancient Indian Contributions to Psychotherapy

Ancient Indian texts offer profound insights into human psychology and mental health. The Vedas, Upanishads, and texts like the Bhagavad Gita provide frameworks for understanding emotions, cognition, and behaviour. Concepts such as '*chitta*' or the mind, '*manas*' or the mental faculty, and '*vikalpa*', the cognitive distortions reflect an intricate understanding of mental processes. Moreover, therapeutic techniques, such as meditation, self-inquiry (*atma-vichara*), and yoga, as described in

S. Halder et al., *Navigating AI in Mental Health Care*,
https://doi.org/10.1007/978-981-96-9744-1_10

Patanjali's Yoga Sutras, laid the groundwork for approaches akin to modern cognitive and behavioural therapies. The dialogues between Krishna and Arjuna in the Bhagavad Gita, for instance, can be interpreted as an early form of cognitive restructuring, where a mentor helps a distressed individual reframe their perspective to find clarity and purpose.

From Philosophy to Science: The Birth of Modern Psychotherapy
As time progressed, these ancient practices influenced philosophical traditions worldwide. However, the formalization of psychotherapy as a discipline began in the late nineteenth century with the development of the most popular form of psychotherapy, psychoanalysis by Freud. Subsequent advancements, including humanistic approach, or behaviourism, and most recent Aaron Beck's cognitive therapy, enriched the field further.

In recent decades, psychotherapy has embraced technology, integrating tools such as online counselling platforms, virtual reality, and artificial intelligence (AI) to address mental health challenges. These innovations draw on both ancient wisdom and modern science, symbolizing the confluence of tradition and progress.

Redefining Mental Health Diagnoses with AI

The traditional framework for diagnosing mental health disorders is largely based on the Diagnostic and Statistical Manual of Mental Disorders (DSM) or the International Classification of Diseases (ICD). However, these classificatory systems rely heavily on symptom-based criteria, which can be subjective and variable. AI offers a transformative, data-driven approach to redefining mental health interventions, addressing the limitations of traditional symptom-based frameworks like the DSM-5. By analysing large datasets, AI identifies biomarkers and subtypes of disorders, enabling precise and personalized diagnostics. For instance, a clinician might use AI tools to identify neuroimaging markers linked to depression, providing a biologically informed diagnosis. AI also excels in early detection, such as spotting prodromal signs of schizophrenia through behavioural patterns, allowing for timely interventions. Predictive models assess risks based on genetic and environmental factors, guiding preventive strategies like counselling for at-risk individuals. Moreover, AI-powered Decision Support Systems (DSS) streamline data integration, automate screening, and suggest evidence-based treatments tailored to unique profiles. For example, an AI system could recommend CBT and mindfulness techniques for an anxiety patient based on their clinical records, ensuring targeted and effective care. These tools support mental health professionals in planning interventions while preserving the critical human element in therapy. Thus, AI needs to be looked at as an assistive companion widening the perspectives human professionals look at, while dealing with patients with mental health care. But yes, the speculations will be there. Professionals might look at AI-based tools as distractions, and a growing tendency to incline on them as a risk of sidelining human clinical expertise.

AI-Driven Cognitive-Behavioural Therapy (CBT)

As we spoke about Cognitive behaviour therapy (CBT) in the opening section, and CBT being one of the most evidence-based psychotherapeutic techniques, it is very much warranted that AI-based therapeutic interventions need to be based on CBT principles. The simplistic nature of the CBT process also makes it suitable to be incorporated in AI-based applications. AI-powered applications can deliver CBT exercises, such as thought challenging and exposure exercises, in a digital format. These tools can reinforce learning and provide consistent support between therapy sessions, helping individuals practice and internalize therapeutic techniques. However, the therapist, and the AI application must be in sync or the application must be vetted by the therapist.

While we speak of the scopes of AI in a positive sense, the patient might have a different inclination for engaging in technology-based interventions and more comfortable with person-to-person interactions. Thus, selection of patients for AI-based intervention also needs to be checked to reduce risk of treatment failure. AI-based applications like Adaptive Treatment Strategies warn therapists of patients at risk of treatment failure to prompt an adaptation of the intervention (Kaldo et al., 2021). It serves as a proactive approach to prevent treatment failure by identifying patients who are not responding well to standard interventions. These strategies use early warning signs—such as lack of improvement in symptoms or engagement—to prompt therapists to adjust the intervention, tailoring it to the patient's unique needs. They are particularly beneficial in context of Internet-delivered Cognitive-Behavioural Therapy (ICBT), which often track patient progress through online questionnaires, symptom monitoring, and behavioural metrics such as completion rates and engagement with therapeutic content. For instance, if a patient shows minimal progress in reducing anxiety or depression levels, ICBT platforms can signal therapists to increase contact frequency or introduce supplementary therapeutic modules. This allows for a more dynamic and responsive treatment process, optimizing outcomes while reducing the risk of patients becoming discouraged by lack of progress. Based on this data, Adaptive Treatment Strategies can suggest real-time adjustments, such as increasing therapist support or modifying the therapy approach if a patient is flagged as being at risk for treatment failure. Thus, applications like these can be particularly useful in preventing dropout or disengagement from therapy, ensuring more personalized care for individuals who may need more intensive or alternative methods of treatment. The support from Adaptive Treatment Strategies enables therapists to deliver support at varying levels such as, **Stepped-care models**, where they start with lower-intensity interventions and step up if required; then **Personalized feedback loops,** helping tailoring therapy content based on individual responses; and **Enhanced therapist engagement,** which adjusts the level of therapist interaction, from automated feedback to more personalized, direct support.

Other Technologies

Neurofeedback and Brain Computer Interface: Even before AI came into prominence, therapists have been using technologies like neurofeedback, and other systems providing interface between human brain and computers. Thus, either way we rely on these technologies and there is no doubt over their reliability as well as utility. EEG (electroencephalography) devices provide feedback to individuals on their brain activity. By training individuals to alter their brainwave patterns, neurofeedback can be used to treat conditions such as ADHD, anxiety, and depression. AI is taking this utility a step further when the algorithms analyse real-time data and compare with existing large datasets to see patterns which experts might miss from their naked eye. Similarly, the brain computer interface has been particularly implicated for emotion regulation, as it allows individuals to interact with computers using their brain signals, providing new ways to practice emotion regulation and self-control. For example, guiding a user through a relaxation exercise by monitoring their brain activity and providing feedback based on their level of arousal. Augmenting AI into existing systems of brain computer interface, may give real-time on spot tasks suitable to the patients. The interventions need not look threatening, as AI-powered therapeutic games that incorporate neurofeedback can make mental health interventions more engaging. For instance, a game might challenge users to maintain a calm state to progress, helping them practice relaxation techniques in a fun and interactive way.

Virtual Reality (VR) and Augmented Reality (AR) Therapies

In previous chapters, we discussed the role of Virtual Reality (VR) and Augmented Reality (AR) therapies emerging as innovative tools to address various mental and physical health challenges. The scope is pretty huge for conditions like different forms of phobia as well as in daily life support for elderly people. These technologies create immersive environments that positively affect brain function, behaviour, mood, and perception. One of the primary advantages of VR is its ability to simulate real-life scenarios, making it an effective tool for treating conditions like phobias, addictions, and anxiety disorders. For example, when a person is in a state of distress or abnormal psychological functioning, VR can immerse them in a controlled virtual environment designed to help them confront their fears or manage their anxiety in a safe and therapeutic manner. By exposing patients to virtual environments tailored to their specific conditions, clinicians can assess and treat the levels of stress, anxiety, or phobia more effectively. Additionally, the use of VR in therapy offers a hands-on, experiential form of treatment, which has been shown to produce significant improvements in mood regulation and behaviour modification. This immersive interaction helps patients rewire their thought processes and reactions to triggering situations.

One of the commonly used techniques in exposure therapy involves the Subjective Unit of Distress Scale (SUD). Developed by Joseph Wolpe in 1969, the assessment is vital in getting a subjective rating of the patient regarding his distress levels on a scale of 0 to 10 for a particular phobic or anxiety provoking situation. Therapists often use SUD in graded exposure to let patients gain improved control and lesser distress in a particular situation, combined with relaxation training. For example, in an imaginal exposure session with a patient having a phobia of dogs, it might be difficult to navigate how the client imagines them in a graded level of proximity to him and if actually he is countering them. However, using VR can make the session more interactive and customizable with better control of the therapist (Fig. 10.1).

Further for elderly individuals facing loneliness, isolation, and physical limitations, maintaining functional autonomy is crucial, as regular physical activity (PA) has been shown to improve health outcomes, reduce the risk of falls, and enhance cognitive functions such as memory and executive function. VR and AR offer immersive and interactive experiences, allowing older adults to engage in simulated environments that promote both physical and mental well-being. VR settings can simulate real-world activities, offering immediate feedback, which is essential for learning and rehabilitation (Manera et al., 2016). These technologies can be personalized to the needs of each individual, making them particularly useful for elderly patients who require tailored interventions.

However, it could be too early to comment, when we can see these technologies in large-scale use among the general public apart from entertainment purposes.

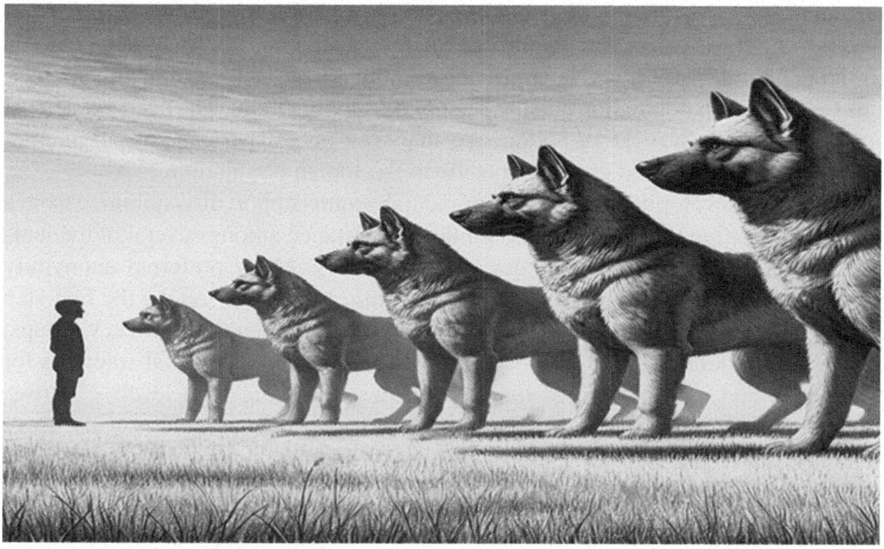

Fig. 10.1 Hypothetical representation of use of VR in imaginal exposure. AI-generated image created with OpenAI, (DALL.E 3, 2024)

Natural Language Processing and Chatbots: The Challenges

We also discussed Natural Language Processing (NLP) in previous chapters as one of the basic elements of AI that focuses on the interaction between computers and human language. NLP has significant applications in mental health, particularly in the development of chatbots and virtual therapists. However, AI applications have been criticized for their limitations of understanding the nuances of human language when spoken in different contexts and sarcasm. While NLP is at the core for understanding the distress of the chatbot user, his health needs as well as understanding a situation if qualifying for an emergency, it also implies a very less margin of error. Even though this issue is being attempted through large databases, one limitation could still linger, whether it can also navigate the cultural contexts and risks of one AI-based application be irrelevant for people from different cultures.

The Experience of Developing CBT-Based Chatbot

The awareness regarding mental health has increased in recent times and particularly after the COVID-19 period, the need for digital form of psychotherapy has heightened. The Indian population has gradually opened up to psychotherapy and cognitive behaviour therapy is one of the popular psychotherapeutic approaches among practising psychologists. However, from our own clinical experience, we have repeatedly felt the gap in terms of non-availability of reliable AI-based mental health applications for the Indian population and the need of developing them. The need got a boost further during the COVID-19 period. We share our own experience of our attempt to develop an AI-powered chatbot, specific to the Indian population.

The idea of developing the chatbot for mental health support also stemmed from a growing realization that there was a significant resistance among several individuals with severe mental health challenges to seek therapy. Many preferred anonymity over face-to-face interactions, and some were entirely hesitant to take the first step towards traditional therapy. With this problem in mind, we identified two key groups: the younger population aged 18–25 years, who often turned to digital solutions for their needs, and working professionals who, despite facing high levels of stress, were reluctant to seek therapy due to stigma or lack of time. Additionally, there was a notable opportunity of using innovative techniques like virtual reality-based exposure therapy in applicable conditions (Fig. 10.2).

Initial Phase: The initial phase was about defining clear objectives. The primary goal was straightforward yet ambitious: to create a chatbot capable of providing basic, anonymous counselling based on Cognitive-Behavioural Therapy (CBT) techniques. This would act as a bridge, encouraging users to seek professional help after their initial interaction. Beyond this, we envisioned a platform that could bring CBT professionals together, introduce VR-based exposure therapy into the Indian market, and promote CBT as a viable solution to mental health challenges.

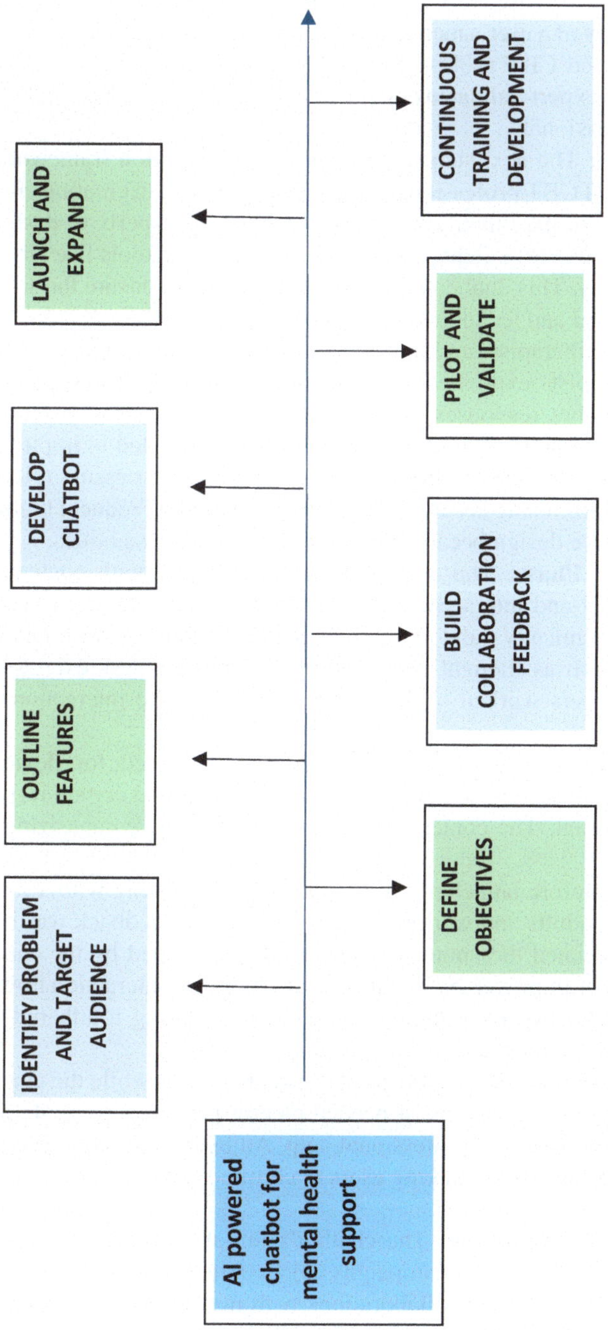

Fig. 10.2 Stepwise framework for developing AI-powered mental health chatbot

Chatbot's Features: We outlined the chatbot's core functionalities, starting with anonymous counselling based on CBT interventions. It would include screening tools to gauge the severity of a user's mental health concerns and a referral system to guide users towards trained CBT professionals. Over time, we planned to expand these features to include expert-validated content, mental health resources, and workshops for users and professionals.

Collaborations: The next step was to build a collaboration framework. On the one side, we needed CBT professionals to provide expertise in creating credible and effective content. On the other, we required technology experts to design a user-friendly, culturally sensitive chatbot, and integrate advanced tools like virtual reality for exposure therapy. This dual collaboration was pivotal to ensure the solution was both clinically sound and technologically robust.

Challenges: As therapists and developers began to work together, they faced a few hurdles. Therapists expressed concerns about oversimplifying complex CBT techniques for chatbot responses. They emphasized the need to balance clinical depth with user-friendliness. Developers, meanwhile, struggled to implement these nuanced techniques into the chatbot's Natural Language Processing (NLP) framework without compromising accuracy or cultural sensitivity. Frequent brainstorming sessions and iterative design became the norm to address these issues.

Developmental Phase: The development phase began with content creation. Screening materials and interactive questionnaires were meticulously designed to ensure they were clinically valid yet approachable. Responses were tailored using CBT principles such as thought restructuring and mindfulness exercises. At the same time, developers worked on integrating NLP to make interactions intuitive and natural.

One key lesson learned during this stage was the need for flexibility. For instance, early user tests revealed that some individuals found certain responses too generic or impersonal. The content was refined repeatedly, emphasizing empathy and relatability.

Pilot Testing: Before launching, we conducted pilot testing with a focus group comprising young adults and working professionals. The feedback was invaluable. While users appreciated the anonymity and guidance offered by the chatbot, they pointed out areas for improvement in the user interface and interaction flow. Concurrently, mental health experts validated the content, ensuring it adhered to ethical guidelines and CBT principles.

Addressing Setbacks: During the pilot, we realized that while the chatbot could effectively address mild concerns, it needed clearer pathways to guide users with severe mental health issues to professional help. Adjustments were made to include a more robust referral system, linking users to certified CBT practitioners and crisis helplines.

Launching and Expanding: The chatbot's initial launch focused on its core counselling features. Marketing campaigns targeted the young and working population through social media and collaborations with mental health organizations. As user engagement grew, we started integrating VR-based exposure therapy solutions for specific phobias, making the platform truly innovative in the Indian context.

Continuous Training: To ensure the platform remained credible and effective, we collaborated with mental health organizations like Indian Association of Cognitive Behaviour Therapy (IACBT). Training modules and workshops were introduced for CBT practitioners, enabling them to utilize the chatbot as a tool to complement their therapy sessions. Feedback loops with both users and professionals became a cornerstone of our approach, ensuring continuous improvement.

In summary, it can be said that the journey was one of learning and adaptation. From understanding the diverse needs of our target audience to addressing technical and ethical challenges, every step contributed to a solution that blended clinical expertise with technological innovation. Today, the chatbot stands not just as a digital tool but as a bridge, empowering individuals to take their first step towards better mental health while advocating for the widespread adoption of CBT.

Some of the Representative Questions Meant to Explore Emotions like Anxiety/Depression Included

How are you feeling today?
What prompted you to reach out?
Can you describe your mood or thoughts recently (e.g. low, anxious, worried)?
Have any recent events in your life affected how you're feeling now?
Has your sleep, appetite, or energy changed recently?
How long have you been feeling this way?
Has this impacted your daily life or routines?
Have you talked to anyone about how you're feeling, or considered seeking professional help?

Now Similar Set of Questions to Set in Chatbot Format Were Like

- *How you are feeling today:*
- *Do you want to share with me anything*
- *You can talk to me anytime*
- *Tell me, if you have any concerns*
- *you mentioned few concerns*
- *Would you like to visit a professional for your problems*

Now, fitting these statements into a chatbot required further modifications. The idea was to make the bot appear friendly, non-judgemental, ready to help, as well as technically sound, and the flow of communication came like this:

Q1 Tell me how are you feeling today? Select smileys from emoji (5 emoji options from very happy to very sad, where emoji 1 is very happy, emoji 2 is quite happy, emoji 3 is neutral, emoji 4 is sad, emoji 5 is very sad).

If emoji 1 or 2 selected, ask Q2. Else go to Q4.

Q 2 I see that you are happy. That's really good to know. However, do you want to share with me anything?

Yes/No. If No, go to Q3, if Yes, go to Q4

Q 3 Great. I am your virtual friend, 24X7. You can talk to me anytime. See you around

Q 4. Could you tell me if you have any concerns which are important to you and which you would like to share with me. I am your virtual friend. Let me reassure you that whatever you share with me remains absolutely confidential. Please select ONLY ONE problem that you may be facing from the list below

Problems: 1. "I am depressed/feel low", 2. "I feel anxious/worried", 3. "I am having personal relationship issues", 4. "I am having a lot of stress at work", 5. "I have self esteem issues", 6. "I feel lonely", 7. "I am having physical health issues", 8. "I have anger issues", 9. "I have phobias", 10. "I am having mood swings", 11. "I am having problems due to my sexual orientation"'

(If more than one problem stated)

Q 5 You have mentioned the following (----------------). Could you please select the most important one from the list

Q6 Would you like to seek any professional help due to this problem? We have a list of very professional counselors/mental healthcare who can help you cope with the problem. I can help you fix an appointment. Would you like to seek an appointment?

Yes/No, If yes, go to Q25, else go to relevant problem selected by person in Q5

"I am depressed/feel low"

1. *Regarding the problem you are facing, how would you describe your predominant mood and thoughts these days? (eg. Low mood, anxious, worried, irritability, nervous, no joy in daily activities etc). Tell me everything you want to talk about. I am your Bestie and I am all ears for you*

Challenges faced: Developing mental health chatbots faces challenges in syncing diverse priorities among mental health professionals, AI experts, and business developers. Effective solutions include interdisciplinary workshops, clear communication channels, and user-centred design to align goals and address concerns effectively.

Missing Empathy in AI Intervention

Empathy and emotional understanding from a psychotherapist are at the heart of effective therapy, creating a safe space where clients feel truly seen and heard. It's not just about listening but about deeply connecting with the client's feelings, struggles, and perspectives. When therapists show genuine care and compassion, clients often describe it as a sense of being "finally understood" or "not judged", which can be transformative. In therapeutic context empathy can be categorized into different types, such as Cognitive empathy: the ability to understand what another person is thinking; emotional empathy: the ability to feel what another person is experiencing emotionally; and compassionate empathy: the ability to not only understand and feel another person's emotions but also to take action to help. This emotional connection fosters trust, encourages openness, and lays the foundation for meaningful growth and healing. Without it, even the best techniques can feel hollow or mechanical.

AI's empathic capabilities are largely limited to cognitive empathy, as it can recognize patterns in language that suggest distress or confusion and respond appropriately. However, it lacks emotional and compassionate empathy because it cannot genuinely experience emotions or take context-driven actions based on a deep understanding of a client's emotional landscape. Human therapists, on the other hand, can integrate all three forms of empathy, which leads to a more holistic and compassionate therapeutic experience.

When Empathy Is Most Needed in Therapy? From a therapeutic methodology perspective, the need for human empathy is especially pronounced in approaches that emphasize the therapeutic relationship, such as psychodynamic therapy, humanistic therapy, and trauma-focused interventions. In these cases, the bond between therapist and client is foundational, and the healing process depends on a deep level of trust and emotional attunement. Conversely, in structured, solution-focused approaches like CBT or behavioural interventions, AI can often substitute for human therapists when the focus is more on the cognitive and behavioural aspects rather than on deep emotional processing. From the patient's perspective, the need for empathy varies based on individual objectives. Some patients may seek therapy primarily for problem-solving or skills-building, where AI's capacity for cognitive empathy and structured guidance may be sufficient. However, others who come to therapy seeking emotional support, validation, or the resolution of complex interpersonal dynamics are likely to benefit far more from the empathic presence of a human therapist. Patients in acute emotional distress, dealing with severe mental health conditions, or navigating crises will also require the warmth and attunement that only human empathy can provide.

While AI can simulate certain aspects of empathic dialogue—such as recognizing and responding to distress or using supportive language—it lacks the depth of emotional resonance that humans naturally offer. AI's responses are algorithmic and data-driven, meaning that the subtleties of human emotions, body language, tone, and shared lived experiences are beyond its current capabilities. In many therapeutic settings, especially those dealing with trauma, grief, or complex mental health issues, the patient's need for authentic human connection cannot be understated. Human therapists provide a unique emotional presence and the ability to understand and connect with clients on an intuitive level. Empathy in therapy is not just about saying the right thing; it is about conveying warmth, trustworthiness, and unconditional positive regard, which are critical for building a therapeutic alliance. This alliance fosters safety, which is essential for patients to explore vulnerable emotions and experiences. Human empathy also involves the ability to read non-verbal cues and adapt one's approach in real-time based on the patient's emotional state.

Empathy can be embedded by training the AI on diverse datasets representing emotional expressions and distress scenarios, enabling it to generate compassionate and validating responses. Regular updates informed by feedback from mental health professionals and users will ensure that the tool remains responsive, culturally sensitive, and aligned with therapeutic best practices, creating a supportive and motivating digital therapy environment.

Balancing AI and Human Empathy: The goal in integrating AI into mental health care should not be to replace human therapists entirely but to complement their work. AI can be a valuable tool in expanding access to care, especially for those who face barriers such as cost, time, or geographical limitations. However, the therapeutic community must remain mindful of the limitations of AI when it comes to empathy and human connection. Further investigation is needed to determine how AI and human therapists can work together in a blended care model that leverages the strengths of both. As AI becomes increasingly sophisticated, it is essential for practitioners and scholars to consider how to best integrate these tools while preserving the core elements of empathy and human connection that are at the heart of effective therapy.

Psychological Intervention for Well-Being

It would be unfair if we focus on psychological interventions with AI for intervention of mental ill health conditions only. Focus should be on overall well-being and wellness of individuals. For that, integrating continuous motivation and empathy into an AI-based psychotherapy tool is very much needed.

It requires a multifaceted approach that combines advanced machine learning algorithms with human-centric design principles. The tools are already using natural language processing (NLP) to detect and respond to the user's emotional tone, context, and progress over time, ensuring tailored support that resonates with their psychological state. Further, by employing reinforcement learning, the AI can adapt its motivational strategies, such as offering personalized encouragement, celebrating milestones, or suggesting achievable goals to sustain user engagement. As more evidence of biomarkers in identifying predispositions of an individual for developing psychopathological symptoms, and early relapse, AI applications can focus on preventive measures like sleep hygiene, managing stress, positive social interactions, physical fitness, cardiac health to name a few which enhance quality of life in general and well-being and also play a role in preventing mental health issues.

Way Forward

AI is transforming psychotherapy by enhancing accessibility, personalization, and scalability, with promising future directions including deeper integration with neural and behavioural data for precision therapy. The main types of AI interventions include chatbots, which simulate therapeutic conversations, and algorithms for symptom monitoring, cognitive restructuring, and emotion recognition, all of which work by leveraging natural language processing and machine learning. These interventions have shown moderate to high efficacy in managing depression and anxiety disorders, often complementing traditional therapy by providing round-the-clock support and tailored strategies. However, challenges such as ensuring data privacy, addressing algorithmic biases, and maintaining human empathy in care highlight the ethical complexities that must be navigated as AI continues to evolve in this field.

Integrating AI into healthcare presents challenges such as automation bias, over-reliance on AI by clinicians, and limited generalizability across diverse populations. Speed-focused AI models may compromise accuracy for certain patients, and the role of visual explanations in identifying biases and supporting decision-making remains uncertain. Effective integration requires a deeper understanding of human-AI interactions, fostering trust, and improving AI literacy among healthcare professionals and patients to ensure reliable and equitable outcomes.

We are now at a point where AI tools can analyse speech patterns, facial expressions, and other subtle non-verbal cues constantly conveyed during virtual therapy sessions. Combined with advancements in generative AI, lifelike avatars, and realistic voice overs, the idea of a fully AI-driven "therapist" is no longer far-fetched. Such a system could potentially read facial expressions, interpret non-verbal signals, converse naturally, and respond in real-time. This raises pressing questions about the future of our profession—questions without clear answers but that demand open dialogue. AI represents an Event Horizon, not only for counselling and psychotherapy but for society as a whole. It will require collective effort to ensure that therapy remains deeply human and to educate clients about the profound relational dynamics that go beyond merely receiving scripted responses.

The essence of therapy lies in its relational risk and reward—the vulnerability of being truly seen and the transformative power of receiving unconditional positive regard from another person, not a programmed entity. The risk of rejection, and the healing that comes when it is replaced by acceptance, is vital to the therapeutic process. A robot that cannot take offence or form an opinion lacks the ability to affirm your inherent worth as a person in the same meaningful way. Without this dynamic, AI-driven interventions may fail to deliver the profound, human-centred outcomes we expect from therapy.

The therapeutic landscape is undoubtedly poised for significant change as AI capabilities grow, promising innovations and efficiencies that could redefine our profession. However, it is essential to remember that the heart of therapy lies in the uniquely human connection—a space defined by empathy, compassion, and shared understanding. Our role as therapists is not diminished but evolving. Rather than choosing between AI and humanity, we must find a balance where AI serves as a tool to enhance, not replace, the sacred, human-centred space of healing and growth that is central to therapy.

Conclusion

AI has the potential to profoundly impact the intervention and treatment of mental health disorders by enhancing early detection, personalizing treatment, and making mental health care more accessible. From redefining diagnostic criteria to supporting therapeutic interventions, AI offers innovative solutions to some of the most pressing challenges in mental health care. However, the successful integration of AI into this field requires careful consideration of ethical issues, robust data protection measures, and a commitment to ensuring that AI technologies are developed and used in ways that promote equity, transparency, and trust. The fundamental question revolves around the balance between the benefits of AI, such as its accessibility and scalability, and the irreplaceable value of human connection, especially when it comes to empathy and the emotional nuances central to effective therapy. AI-based applications also need to be reliable in navigating cultural barriers and language nuances, and at the same time be cost effective to all stakeholders. By addressing these challenges, AI can become a powerful tool for improving mental health outcomes and transforming the way mental health care is delivered.

References

Kaldo, V., Isacsson, N., Forsell, E., Bjurner, P., Abdesslem, F. B., & Boman, M. (2021). AI-driven adaptive treatment strategies in internet-delivered CBT. *European Psychiatry, 64*(Suppl 1), S20. https://doi.org/10.1192/j.eurpsy.2021.75

Manera, V., Chapoulie, E., Bourgeois, J., Guerchouche, R., David, R., Ondrej, J., et al. (2016). A feasibility study with image-based rendered virtual reality in patients with mild cognitive impairment and dementia. *PLoS ONE, 11*(3), e0151487. https://doi.org/10.1371/journal.pone.0151487

OpenAI. (2024). *A humorous cartoon illustration depicting two psychotherapists discussing AI.* DALL·E. Generated on December 1, 2024.

Wolpe, J. (1969). *The practice of behavior therapy.* Pergamon Press, ISBN 0080065635.

Chapter 11
AI Support for Mental Healthcare Professionals

Abstract Every technology developed impacts its users as well as professionals handling it. While these impacts are generally meant to be positive, at times they are met with apprehensions which are often grounded on limited awareness or misinformation. The chapter throws light on the emerging relation between professionals and AI, the perception of mental health professionals regarding AI, and the scope of improving this emerging relation for improved mental health services. We also highlight the results from a survey that examined mental health professional's opinions on how AI is affecting their jobs, and what they actually expect from AI. The relationship between technology and mental health professionals is thoroughly reviewed, with a focus on collaboration for better patient care. The state of AI in mental health care is examined, along with potential future directions.

Keywords Mental health professionals · Treatment adherence · AI integrated training · Virtual support

Perception and Awareness Regarding AI

AI came into limelight and prominence only a few years back, but its stellar rise is phenomenal to the extent that professionals in different fields even for once, must have pondered how it is going to impact their field. It may be hypothesized that a professional's opinion regarding use of AI depends on his or her awareness of how AI works and its capabilities. Mental health experts are no exception, and if an expert conventionally is asked on his opinion about some of his work to be assisted or shared by AI, the initial string of thoughts may sound like-

- *How could a machine interview a psychiatric patient? It cannot show empathy.*
- *Computers are good. Am already using them for managing appointments. But how can you trust them for therapy? Can you trust them when you are dealing with a suicidal patient? They will sound like monotonous robots with fixed answers, whatever you ask them. They will never match the humane touch and sensitivity. It's ok if you use them for reminders for medicines or session follow up.*

S. Halder et al., *Navigating AI in Mental Health Care*,
https://doi.org/10.1007/978-981-96-9744-1_11

- *Oh, those are fancy engineering stuff and sounds good for reputed research centres in university labs. We are out of it.*
- *Yes, I have seen some of the chatbots. But they are still in trial version. Will they ever come in mass use? How will clinics and hospitals integrate them in their system?* (Fig. 11.1).

Concerns like these are real and expected. We discussed in our preliminary chapter how public opinion about AI differs and this difference was stark between nationals of different countries. While the United States leads the globe in terms of AI research and funding, it is interesting to note that individuals in the United States are more sceptical and concerned about AI, compared to countries like China or India. In similar fashion, mental health experts may have divided opinion on how they look at implications of AI in their field. It is the need of the hour, that all stakeholders in the field of mental health realize the potential of AI for its judicial use.

AI is unlike any other technologies developed before, as it has the capacity to learn and evolve, and in the course requires constant monitoring, so that it remains safe, reliable, and ethical. Though a non-living entity, AI needs to be treated as a companion by professionals, and the process starts with understanding it better.

A professionals' familiarity with AI varies widely. From a mental health professional perspective, the implication or role of AI at present is at different levels depending on infrastructural readiness of the clinic or hospital they are engaged

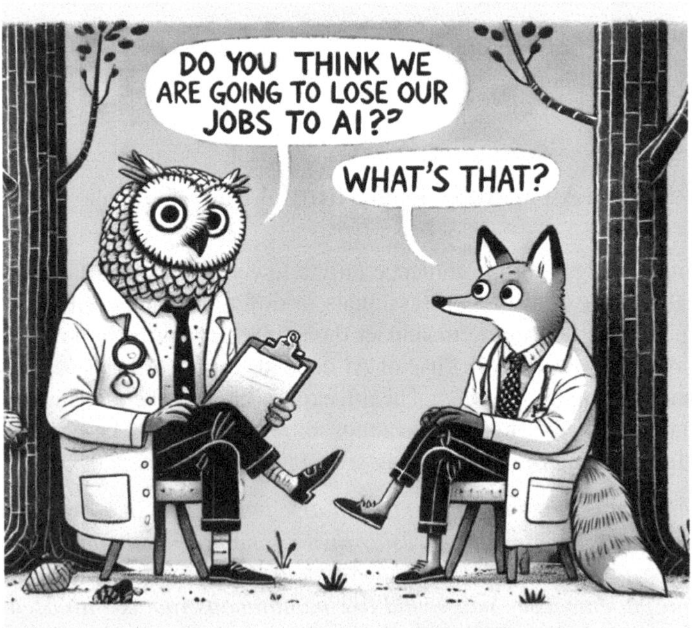

Fig. 11.1 Differences in awareness, attitude, and apprehensions towards AI. *AI-generated image created with OpenAI* (DALL.E 3, 2024)

in, as well as availability of such applications, as well as their own familiarity of AI applications. Some professionals may have a very basic understanding of AI, perceiving it like an online service which gives answers to your queries. Some might be familiar with platforms like OpenAI's ChatGPT or Google's Gemini and use it for minor assistance in their professional work. Others might be aware of the advances happening globally but wondering how it is going to happen, while others might have only encountered the concept in passing and given it little attention. Thus, there appears to be a dilemma whether to board the 'bus' or wait for some time, till the journey is declared to be safe!

We highlight the findings of an online survey conducted by us in the year 2023–24 to explore the opinions of mental health professionals regarding the influence of artificial intelligence (AI) on their jobs. With AI technologies becoming increasingly integrated into various domains, including mental health services, this study aimed to provide insights into the perceptions, challenges, and opportunities associated with AI in this field.

Out of a total of **150 mental health professionals** participating in the survey; psychiatrists constituted 40% of the sample followed by trained psychologists at 35% and counsellors and other mental health professionals at 25%, who were provided with a structured questionnaire (Fig. 11.2).

The survey results showed a satisfactory level of awareness regarding AI in mental health professionals, where psychiatrists responded in highest percentage, followed by trained psychologists and then counsellors.

The qualitative responses from the survey also revealed a high percentage of participants (72%) agreeing on the potential of AI in improving accessibility to mental health care. However, a highly significant number of professionals (42%) saw AI as a threat to job security also, and 20% were concerned about ethical practice of AI usage in mental health (Figs. 11.3 and 11.4).

The participating professionals highlighted the opportunities AI brought in mental health services delivery, but also raised concerns regarding ethical practices, data

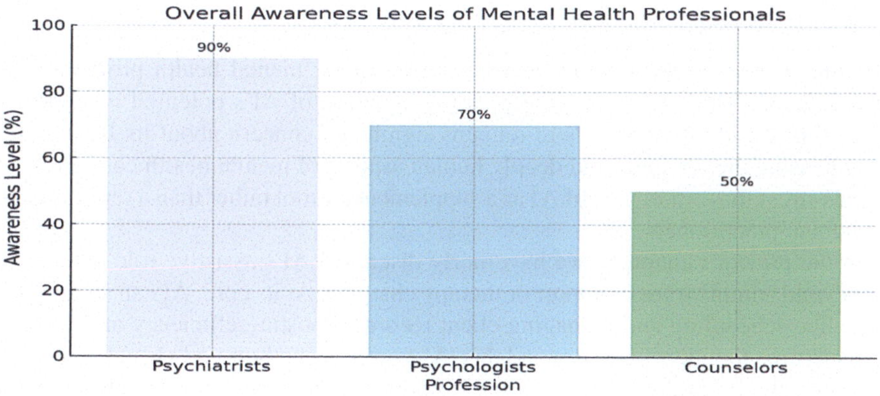

Fig. 11.2 Awareness of different mental health professionals about use of AI in mental health

Question	Agree (%)	Neutral (%)	Disagree (%)
AI tools improve accessibility to mental health care	72%	18%	10%
AI can effectively assist in early diagnosis	65%	22%	13%
AI poses a threat to job security in mental health	28%	30%	42%
Ethical concerns about AI in mental health services	55%	25%	20%
AI will never replace human empathy in therapy	89%	8%	3%

Fig. 11.3 Perception of professionals towards AI

privacy, loss of humane touch in the therapy process, its cost-effectiveness, sensitivity to culture, capability of deciphering language nuances, and so on.

Some verbatim from participating professionals are mentioned below:

- "*I read a lot regarding AI; but do not see it happening very soon. If it is implemented by private providers, it will raise the cost of treatment. This is more suitable for western countries*".
- "*I see AI as an ally, not a threat. It can help with administrative burdens, giving me more time to focus on the therapeutic relationship with my clients*".
- "*May be my knowledge is limited but suppose an AI application is made to assist in the therapy process. So, it has to capture data in terms of the transcript. This will require additional machinery or software, which patients may not like. Also, how will the app understand the exact emotional connotation of the communication*".
- "*There's a risk that younger professionals might become too dependent on AI and lose the art of critical thinking and intuition that's vital in mental health care*".
- "*AI tools must be culturally sensitive. An algorithm trained on one demographic might misinterpret or even harm patients from different backgrounds*".
- "*Some of my clients are already using AI-powered apps for journaling, and it's interesting to see how they feel 'heard,' even by a machine*".
- "*I'd like to see more transparency from developers about how these AI tools actually work and where they're getting their data*".

The findings highlight a nuanced perspective among mental health professionals regarding AI. While there is widespread recognition of AI's potential to improve accessibility and efficiency, there remains significant concern about its limitations in addressing the complex and deeply human aspects of mental health care. Professionals stress the importance of AI as a supplementary tool rather than a replacement for human practitioners.

In the previous chapters, we have fairly discussed AI's assistive role extending far beyond administrative support or therapy chatbots. At its core, AI can streamline tasks like scheduling and managing client records, boosting efficiency and freeing up more time for client care. Beyond this, AI-powered chatbots and virtual assistants are increasingly used to provide initial support and triage, offering a valuable first layer of assistance that benefits both individual practitioners and larger organizations.

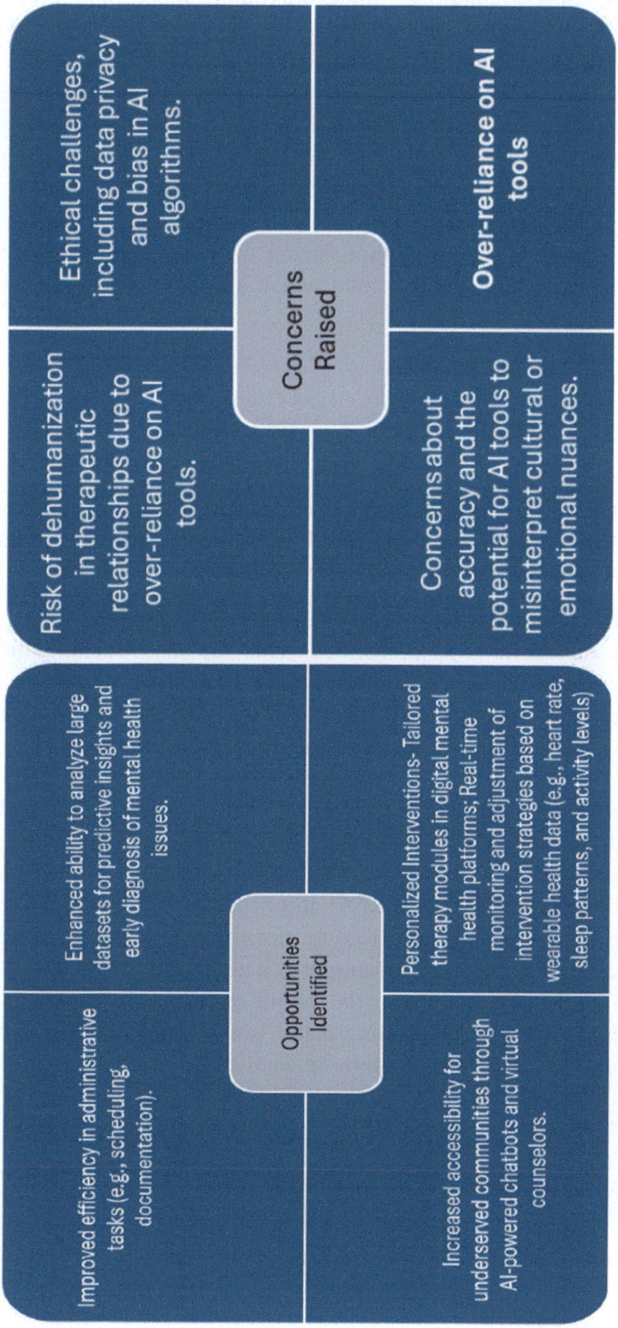

Fig. 11.4 Opportunities and concerns regarding use of AI

Some therapists also leverage generative AI to navigate ethical dilemmas between supervision sessions or to deepen their understanding of theoretical models. Additionally, AI-assisted therapy and chatbots are being employed to offer clients extra support outside of sessions or when therapists are unavailable.

This intersection of artificial intelligence (AI) and mental healthcare presents a transformative potential to reshape the way professionals engage with individuals facing mental health challenges. By leveraging AI, mental healthcare providers can offer more personalized, accessible, and proactive care, effectively guiding individuals through their recovery journey. This elaboration explores various AI-driven client engagement strategies, emphasizing their applications, benefits, and implications for mental health management which all stakeholders must be aware of.

AI Integration in Mobile Health Applications

Mobile health applications, commonly referred to as mHealth apps, have become increasingly popular as tools for mental health management. AI can be seamlessly integrated into these platforms to support individuals in several ways:

- **Medication Management**: AI can send personalized reminders to users, ensuring they take their medications as prescribed. This includes tracking the timing, dosage, and frequency of medication intake. For individuals managing complex medication regimens, AI can reduce the cognitive load associated with remembering medication schedules. Wearable devices and mobile applications can track behavioural and physiological data (like sleep, heart rate, or activity levels) in real-time, providing insights into a patient's mental state between sessions. Learning to work with these AI-enabled monitoring systems can help clinicians enhance their understanding of patient progress and adjust treatments accordingly.
- **Adherence Tracking and Feedback**: AI algorithms can analyse adherence data and provide feedback to users, reinforcing positive behaviours and addressing potential barriers to adherence. For example, if a user consistently misses evening doses, the app might suggest adjusting the routine or provide motivational support.
- **Side Effect Monitoring**: By collecting data from users about their experiences with medications, AI can identify patterns and correlations between specific drugs and adverse effects. This real-time monitoring enables healthcare providers to make timely adjustments to treatment plans, improving patient safety and comfort.
- **Healthcare Collaboration**: AI-driven platforms can facilitate communication between patients and healthcare providers by automatically sharing relevant data, such as mood patterns or medication adherence. This promotes a collaborative approach to care, where healthcare providers can make more informed decisions based on real-time information.

Mood Monitoring and Trigger Identification

AI technologies can monitor mood fluctuations by analysing data from various sources, such as self-reported mood logs, sensor data, and even natural language processing of user input. This continuous monitoring offers several advantages:

- **Pattern Recognition**: AI can identify patterns in mood changes and correlate them with specific triggers, such as changes in sleep patterns, social interactions, or environmental factors. Understanding these patterns enables individuals to make proactive decisions about their self-care, such as avoiding known triggers or implementing coping strategies during vulnerable times.
- **Personalized Interventions**: Based on the identified patterns, AI can suggest personalized interventions, such as mindfulness exercises, physical activities, or reaching out to a support network. This tailored approach enhances the relevance and effectiveness of the recommendations.
- **Predictive Analytics**: By analysing historical data, AI can predict potential mood changes and alert users and their healthcare providers before significant mood episodes occur. This predictive capability is particularly valuable for individuals with conditions like bipolar disorder, where early intervention can prevent severe mood swings.

Enhancing Therapeutic Engagement

AI can enhance therapeutic engagement by providing continuous support and reinforcement outside of traditional therapy sessions:

- **Virtual Support Agents**: AI-driven chatbots and virtual agents can offer immediate support to users, providing coping strategies, psychoeducation, or simply a listening ear. These agents are available 24/7, offering an accessible resource for individuals in distress. However, one possible pitfall could be that these virtual agents need to be vetted by the therapist and also agreed upon by the patient. In event, these are not in-house development, it could add extra cost to the patient.
- **Progress Tracking and Feedback**: AI applications can track an individual's progress over time, providing feedback on their efforts and celebrating milestones. For example, an app might congratulate a user for completing a week of mindfulness practice, reinforcing positive behaviours and boosting motivation.
- **Personalized Content Delivery**: AI can curate personalized content, such as articles, videos, or exercises, based on an individual's preferences and progress. This tailored approach ensures that users receive relevant and engaging materials that support their therapeutic journey. It could be very beneficial for patients with substance abuse trying to be sober and struggling with controlling their impulses.

Informal Use of Smart Technology and Social Networking Among Healthcare Professionals

Even though AI is yet to make fill fledged inroads to mental health services, professionals already have been using smart technologies. The use of social networking apps has become increasingly important among healthcare professionals, transforming how they communicate, collaborate, and share knowledge. These apps, including general platforms such as WhatsApp, Facebook, and LinkedIn, as well as healthcare-specific ones like 'Doximity' and 'Fig. 11.1', offer versatile tools for professional engagement. Social networking apps enable professionals to connect with peers, seek advice on clinical cases, and share knowledge in real-time. For instance, WhatsApp groups are frequently used by physicians, nurses, and allied health workers to discuss patient cases, exchange best practices, and provide mutual support, especially in rural or resource-limited settings. Platforms like Fig. 11.1 allow professionals to share anonymized patient images and receive input from a global network of experts, fostering collaborative problem-solving and continuous learning. These capabilities enhance not only individual skillsets but also team-based care, ultimately improving patient outcomes. Despite these benefits, there are several challenges associated with the use of social networking apps in healthcare. A primary concern is data privacy and security, as the exchange of sensitive patient information over these platforms can expose healthcare providers to legal and ethical risks. Many apps lack end-to-end encryption, which raises questions about the protection of patient confidentiality. Additionally, the blending of professional and personal use on social media can blur boundaries, leading to potential breaches of professionalism. Professionals must navigate these risks carefully by adhering to guidelines and ensuring that apps are used responsibly. Another issue is the potential for misinformation to spread through social networks. While these apps provide a means to share evidence-based information, they can also amplify inaccurate or unverified content. Health professionals are increasingly tasked with addressing this challenge by promoting credible sources and countering harmful narratives. To mitigate these risks, training in digital literacy and the ethical use of social media is essential for healthcare providers.

Mental health professionals generally recognize the potential of AI to augment their practice but express concerns about overreliance on technology. Ethical issues, such as data privacy and bias in AI algorithms, are frequently highlighted. Professionals emphasize the need for robust safeguards to ensure that AI tools are accurate, culturally sensitive, and ethically deployed. Thus, training be it formal or self-learned appear to be becoming vital for integration of AI into clinical practice. While some practitioners are enthusiastic about using AI for patient assessment and treatment planning, others feel inadequately prepared to incorporate these technologies. Continuous education and collaboration with AI developers are crucial to bridging this gap.

Training

While the scope of AI in mental health gets bigger with every passing day; access to credible applications and familiarity as well as competency of professionals over these applications is an issue which aptly requires orientation and training of professionals for proper and adequate use of AI in practice. As the use of AI in mental health care offers many benefits, it also raises important ethical considerations. Healthcare professionals must ensure that the use of AI is consistent with ethical standards and that patient privacy and confidentiality are protected. Additionally, healthcare professionals must be mindful of the limitations of AI and not rely solely on AI algorithms for making important treatment decisions.

The application of the AI-based techniques could be very basic in nature like taking appointments to advanced levels like identifying biomarkers and potential risk of relapse. Thus, some of the applications might require providing orientation training in the following domains:

- **Multimodal Data Integration**: Future AI systems may integrate data from multiple sources, such as wearable devices, electronic health records, and genetic information, to provide a more comprehensive view of an individual's mental health. This multimodal approach could lead to more accurate assessments and personalized interventions. As health records or genetic information or other information are likely to be from different specialties, it might be tricky for professionals to keep track of them; thus, professionals should have access as well as training to put data from multiple sources for prediction and decision-making.
- **Virtual Reality (VR) and AI**: For many people VR corresponds to immersive video games. But, the integration of AI and VR technology could create immersive therapeutic experiences, such as virtual exposure therapy for anxiety disorders or VR-based social skills training for individuals with autism. Professionals, thus, may be acquainted with the basics of VR and its customization for optimizing therapeutic outcomes with their patients.
- **AI-Driven Screening Tools**: AI-powered screening tools can assess risk factors for conditions like depression, anxiety, or PTSD based on user responses to questionnaires and behavioural data. These tools can be integrated into routine healthcare visits, enabling early identification and referral to appropriate services. Since these screening tools may not be direct questions like paper-pencil-based test and could rely on different markers, professionals also need to adapt them with the new screening techniques.
- **Automated Check-ins**: AI can initiate automated check-ins with users, asking about their well-being and prompting them to engage with supportive resources if needed. This proactive approach ensures that individuals receive ongoing support, even between formal therapy sessions. However, professionals would be required to provide their inputs into the online system which could be different from their conventional offline setup and thus need to be explained the process.
- **Behavioural Change Detection & Emotion Recognition**: AI-based mental health applications can detect subtle changes in behaviour that may precede the

onset of mental health conditions. For example, a sudden decrease in social interactions or a shift in communication style may indicate emerging depressive symptoms. Early detection allows for pre-emptive support, potentially preventing the condition from worsening. However, professionals are not expected to have access to this data, unless patients report to them. Upon reporting, professionals should be aware of the application interface to aid in decision-making about the patient.

- **Bias Reduction and Cultural Sensitivity**: AI systems trained on diverse datasets can help clinicians better understand and accommodate cultural factors in mental health, as some systems are designed to reduce biases. Training in AI applications that support cultural sensitivity can improve inclusivity in mental health care.

Concerns on the Capability

While AI is gearing up to become a handy companion of mental health professionals, the professionals also raise certain valid concerns on the capability of AI in navigating the following domains:

The Need for Culturally Competent AI: Professionals emphasize the importance of cultural competence in mental health interventions. AI tools must be designed to recognize and respect diverse cultural expressions of mental health and distress. This entails incorporating a wide range of linguistic, social, and historical contexts into AI training datasets. Without this, AI risks providing one-size-fits-all solutions that may not resonate with or benefit all patient groups. For instance, understanding the cultural stigma surrounding mental health in some communities is crucial for tailoring interventions. Mental health professionals are therefore advocating for inclusive development processes that involve diverse populations and stakeholders to ensure AI tools are equitable and effective.

Integration Challenges and Training Needs: Integrating AI into clinical practice presents both logistical and professional challenges. While some practitioners are enthusiastic about using AI to streamline patient assessments or identify high-risk cases through predictive analytics, others express concerns about their readiness to do so. This gap highlights a pressing need for comprehensive training programmes to familiarize professionals with AI functionalities and limitations. Moreover, mental health professionals advocate for tools that are user-friendly and seamlessly integrate into existing workflows. If AI systems are too complex or time-consuming to use, they may inadvertently add to the workload rather than alleviate it. Collaboration between AI developers and mental health practitioners is essential to design systems that are both intuitive and clinically meaningful.

Balancing Technology and Human Connection: A recurring theme among professionals is the irreplaceable value of human connection in mental health care. While AI can efficiently handle administrative tasks, provide immediate responses, or support self-guided therapy, it cannot replicate the empathy, warmth, and nuanced understanding of a human therapist. Professionals stress that AI should be viewed as a complement, not a replacement, to human expertise.

For example, AI tools can help gather preliminary information or monitor patient progress, allowing therapists to focus on deeper therapeutic engagement. However, professionals caution against overreliance on AI, which could inadvertently dehumanize care or create a perception that technology can fully substitute for personal interaction.

Professionals' Perspectives on Patients Accessing Electronic Health Records

The increasing use of web-based platforms to grant patients access to their electronic health records has transformed the dynamics of mental health care, prompting mixed reactions from professionals. On one hand, providing patients with direct access to their health information aligns with modern principles of transparency, patient-centred care, and empowerment. Studies have shown that patients who can review their electronic health records are more likely to feel engaged in their treatment, leading to improved communication and collaboration between patients and clinicians. In mental health care specifically, web-based access allows patients to track progress in therapy, revisit recommendations, and gain insights into their diagnoses and treatment plans. This transparency can demystify the therapeutic process, reduce anxiety, and help patients better understand the steps required for their recovery.

However, mental health professionals express valid concerns about the implications of providing unmediated access to sensitive information, such as diagnoses, therapist notes, or test results, which could be misinterpreted or distressing without proper context. For instance, reading clinical terms or assessments intended for internal communication may lead to confusion or emotional distress if not adequately explained by a professional. These concerns are compounded in cases where patients are dealing with severe mental illnesses, such as schizophrenia or borderline personality disorder, where certain information might exacerbate symptoms or lead to distrust between the patient and clinician.

Professionals also highlight the potential for such access to disrupt therapeutic alliances if patients perceive certain entries as overly judgemental or stigmatizing. Furthermore, there are challenges related to the digital divide; not all patients have equal access to the technology or digital literacy required to navigate the health record platforms effectively, potentially widening health disparities. From a technical perspective, mental healthcare professionals stress the importance of user-friendly interfaces and clear language to ensure that the information provided is accessible and understandable.

They also emphasize the need for robust security measures to protect patient privacy, as web-based platforms are vulnerable to breaches that could compromise sensitive data. Ethical dilemmas arise regarding how much information should be shared.

Research also indicates that the success of web-based health record access in mental health care depends on educating both patients and professionals about the system's purpose, limitations, and appropriate use. While some practitioners are hesitant about fully adopting such platforms, they acknowledge that, when implemented thoughtfully, web-based access to health records can enhance trust, improve outcomes, and encourage a collaborative care model.

Ethical and Practical Concerns

One of the most frequently cited concerns among professionals is the ethical deployment of AI tools. The sensitive nature of mental health data amplifies the importance of robust data privacy measures and transparent practices in data collection, storage, and use. Professionals worry about the risk of breaches and misuse, as well as the potential for bias within AI algorithms. For instance, algorithms trained on non-diverse datasets may perpetuate stereotypes or fail to account for cultural, linguistic, and socioeconomic nuances in mental health care. In addition, there are concerns about accountability and liability. Mental health professionals' question who bears responsibility when AI-generated recommendations lead to suboptimal or harmful outcomes. This uncertainty highlights the need for clear legal and ethical frameworks governing the use of AI in clinical settings.

Way Forward for AI Support for Mental Healthcare Professionals

The integration of Artificial Intelligence (AI) in mental healthcare presents a transformative opportunity for mental health professionals. However, there are some challenges which need to overcome by professionals.

- Future demands a strategic approach to foster both awareness and understanding of mental health complexities and AI capabilities.
- Mental health professionals also need to be well-versed in AI technologies, such as diagnostic tools, predictive algorithms, and therapy chatbots, while ensuring these technologies are grounded in evidence-based mental health principles. For example, a clinician utilizing an AI-based screening tool for depression could combine its insights with their clinical judgement to better tailor interventions.
- Research and clinical practice must work hand in hand, exploring ways AI can enhance treatment effectiveness. This includes using AI to identify patterns in large datasets for understanding mental health trends or personalizing therapy based on a client's unique needs, as seen in AI-driven Cognitive-Behavioural Therapy (CBT) apps.
- Equally important is breaking the myths surrounding AI. Some clients might fear that AI will replace therapists or compromise their privacy. Educating clients about AI as a supportive, rather than a replacing, tool is crucial. For instance, a therapist introducing an AI journaling app to a client can explain how it complements therapy by offering daily emotional tracking, while the human therapist provides the relational and empathetic connection that technology cannot replicate.

- Innovations in AI can lead to novel interventions, such as virtual reality exposure therapy or predictive mental health monitoring, but they must not overshadow the human component. A counsellor using AI for preliminary assessments must ensure the therapeutic alliance remains central, as empathy, active listening, and trust cannot be programmed.
- The way forward lies in fostering interdisciplinary collaboration between technologists, clinicians, and researchers, and committing to continuous education, ethical innovation, and a client-centred approach that honours the irreplaceable human connection in psychological care.

Conclusion

AI-driven client engagement strategies offer a powerful toolkit for mental healthcare professionals to support individuals on their recovery journey. The awareness, and perception of mental health professionals towards AI, varies significantly. By leveraging AI for medication management, mood monitoring, early detection, therapeutic engagement, and community building, mental health professionals can provide more personalized, accessible, and effective care. However, the integration of AI in mental health care must be approached with careful consideration of ethical, privacy, and bias issues to ensure safe and equitable outcomes for all users. While mental healthcare professionals raise concerns about potential lack of empathy, humane concern, understanding of cultural and language nuances by AI-based technologies; there is also a need of orienting professionals on scope as well as basics of AI. As technology advances, continued innovation and collaboration between AI researchers and mental health professionals will be essential to unlocking the full potential of AI in mental health care.

Reference

OpenAI. (2024). *A humorous cartoon illustration depicting two psychotherapists discussing AI*. DALL·E. Generated on December 1, 2024.

Chapter 12
Ethical Issues and Considerations for AI

Abstract Data is often termed as the 'new gold'. As Artificial Intelligence (AI) rises in prominence, it essentially feeds on data. This brings an equally important and challenging task of its ethical management and safeguard. There are chances, rather evidences where AI can also make some errors and be biased. The present chapter highlights on the issues of ethical management of data and algorithm bias. We further discuss on transparency in the data management process, security aspects as well as intellectual property. Existing guidelines and legal provisions and acts at present are also discussed.

Keywords Ethical challenges · AI Eco system · Privacy and security · Transparency

Whether My Information Is Safe?

Anushree (name changed) had been an active user of the social media and frequently shared her pictures with her friends. She was excited with her recently bought smartphone and its impressive camera and features to make collages and videos. She got a pleasant surprise when the camera application on its own made a video of compiled pictures of her sister with a nice musical background, and it popped on her screen. She was amused and happy to see the video and instantly shared the same to her sister. But she noticed one thing that made her worried. The video was titled after her sister's name. How could the camera application know her sister's name? She worried, if the app could know her sister's name, what other information it could track. Maybe her worries were genuine, maybe not.

S. Halder et al., *Navigating AI in Mental Health Care*,
https://doi.org/10.1007/978-981-96-9744-1_12

The AI Ecosystem and the Stakeholders

It is a known fact that our online activities are prone to tracking by multiple players, who use the information in different ways, and at times detrimental for the user. So, when we speak of Artificial intelligence and its increasing role in our lives and especially the health sector; how much the AI ecosystem plays by ethical norms.

AI systems are increasingly becoming an integral part of our daily lives, making decisions that directly impact us. From recommending products to diagnosing diseases, these applications are used everywhere. However, a critical question that arises is, do we understand how these technologies work and can we trust these systems? Some may tend to believe that machines making decisions must be accurate and unbiased, however, this may not be absolute truth. To understand the potential pitfalls, the ethical, security, and privacy concerns, we need to understand the inner intricacies involved in designing, building, operating, and using these AI systems and the products embedded with AI technology.

Broadly speaking, there are two components of the AI systems, the *Machine Learning models,* and the *data.* From a people perspective, there are three distinct groups who interact with these systems, the *developers* who build the systems, the *practitioners* who use them, and the *consumers* who are the beneficiary. For example, an AI-enabled healthcare equipment is developed by an organization, with developers building the system and embedding the AI capabilities in the products, the medical practitioners use the systems for diagnosis of diseases and treatment of the patients, and the patients are the consumers, who rely on the doctors, medical practitioners, and the medical systems for their healthcare needs. In some cases, the applications are used directly by users, like the healthcare mobile apps, which have two key stakeholders, the *developers* of the app and the *consumers.* In the mental health domain, there are many apps available in the mobile app stores which are just a click away for anyone with a mobile device to use (Fig. 12.1).

In this ecosystem, each stakeholder has different goals and objectives. The organizations that develop the AI systems or the product manufacturers need to focus

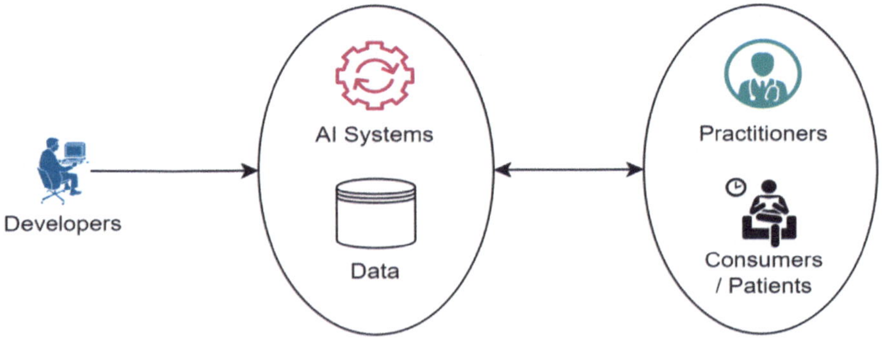

Fig. 12.1 Stakeholders of AI systems

on profitability of the business, research, and innovation for continual enhancement of the systems, business partnerships, marketing and competitive positioning of the products, version releases, after-sales maintenance, and customer support. There are various challenges that need to be addressed to meet the objectives, like innovation, research, faster go-to-market strategies, profitability, cost management, vendor relationships, acquire and retain the talent pool, and so on. The practitioners, i.e., the doctors and the healthcare professionals, need the medical equipment to provide accurate diagnosis and outcomes, which they can rely on for treatment of the patients. The other factors like availability and sustainability of the medical systems are critical for patient care. The reputation of the practitioners is of high stake, which demands the AI systems embedded into the medical equipment to be truly reliable in the results and outcomes they produce. There are regulatory and compliance requirements that need to be adhered to by the product manufacturers and practitioners, as well. The consumers, i.e., the patients and their well-wishers want the best quality treatment at an affordable cost, with no risk of failure. Human rights like dignity, the right to privacy, non-discrimination are inherent expectations of any patient.

Several questions arise, considering the stakeholders with varied objectives and interests.

- *How reliable are the AI systems?*
- *Is the machine learning models within the AI systems inferring correctly?*
- *Have the systems been extensively tested before they are being used in real-world situations?*
- *How relevant is the data on which the machine learning models are trained on?*
- *Is there any risk of data breach for the personal information of the patients?*
- *Who has access to the sensitive medical records of the patients?*
- *How is the personal data being used?*
- *Who is responsible for any negative outcomes arising from these systems?*

To address concerns like these, there are many dimensions that need to be considered for designing, developing, and implementing AI embedded systems, from balancing risk and innovation to decisions concerning security and privacy. In healthcare systems, the stakes are high as it deals with medical conditions of patients, including risk to life. There are several factors that need to be considered in the life cycle of AI systems, as depicted in Fig. 12.2.

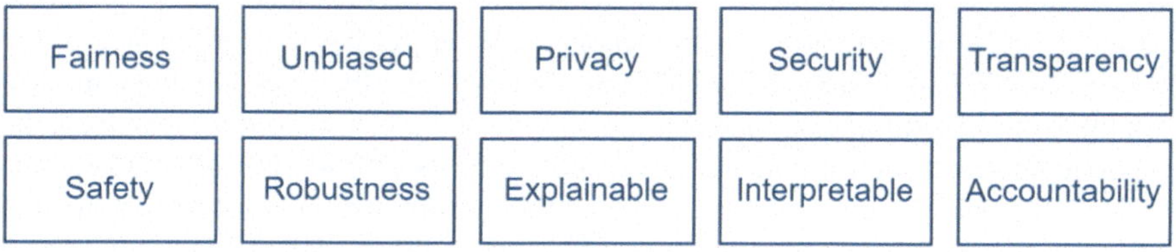

Fig. 12.2 Key considerations for AI systems

Under the hood of the AI systems are the *data* and the *models*. It is crucial to ensure that the data and the models are developed in a way that produces fair results from the systems. Fairness in the systems is essential to ensure that the AI systems do not discriminate against certain groups or individuals. The systems need to be unbiased, however the real world is not so, with a lot of bias ingrained within our society. This influences the design, development, and training of the AI systems, including bias in the data and the way decisions are made in the AI lifecycle from development to deployment.

AI is not just a technological challenge. It is a socio-technological challenge that must be addressed holistically considering all aspects of people, process, and technology. The design and development of AI systems not only need to consider the technical methods and tools, but also the people, culture, diversity, and inclusiveness in the organizations. There are risks of AI systems propagating biased information and discriminating against communities, and these risks need to be addressed before a system may be launched for real-world use. The greater the diversity, the higher the chances of spotting any bias and addressing them before they are released for public use.

The organizations developing the systems are expected to be accountable and responsible for the products they build and deploy. However, with many parties involved this is a complex area to address. Also, AI systems cannot be treated as a black box, even though the underlying neural network models are black-box models. It is crucial to be able to understand how the systems work, especially when these systems are being used in situations that impact human lives. For industries like health care and finance, it is of paramount importance to be able to explain how the models make the decisions and there is a clear understanding of the way the results are to be interpreted.

Data is said to be the new oil and the enormous amount of data that is used for training machine learning models, guide the systems on how it would infer in real-world situations on unseen data. There are various questions that arise on whether there is any bias in the data or even if the data used for training is causing copyright issues. Also, with a significant amount of personal data being handled within the systems how is safety and privacy of the systems being dealt with? Are the systems robust enough to deliver expected results under all circumstances?

Generative AI has brought in a new set of challenges compared to traditional machine learning. Generative AI uses large language models that are trained on huge corpus of data available on the internet. As the models learn from the data it is trained on, these generative AI models provide output based on what was in the training data. When datasets have bias and toxic content, the large language models have the risk of learning from it and producing biased and toxic output which can be detrimental to the need for which it is intended to be used. The generative AI models also have the risk of hallucinating, i.e., providing output, which is not true. When the training data is not sufficient to provide a prediction, the models tend to make up an answer which may be factually incorrect, baseless, and completely imaginary. There are copyright infringement concerns, with many lawsuits being filed by authors, artists, and organizations whose work may have been used for training AI models without their consent.

These concerns lead to the discussion on safety, security, privacy, transparency, and fairness of the AI systems. Usage of AI is the future across industries, and there is no way adoption of AI may be avoided, however there is a need for governance and regulations to manage and mitigate the risks involved. To grapple with these issues, ethics in AI has become a critical point of discussion and research, and businesses are trying to address the ethical challenges through their principles and practices.

In the **healthcare and mental health domain**, AI is increasingly being used in medical systems used for diagnosis and treatment. Medical care devices are not only limited to hospitals and clinics but are now extending to the people as a self-help tool, through wearable devices like smartwatches and mobile apps. All these devices capture health parameters of individuals and can be beneficial in early detection of health problems. AI systems can also predict medical conditions based on various data points and patterns observed in a patient's health parameters, well before the actual problem happens. There are many healthcare and mental health apps and chatbots available for public use, however there are concerns on how the user data collected by these apps are stored, processed, reused, and distributed.

There are questions that come up, like whether the patients' data collected in the process is anonymized and de-identified to prevent identification of individuals? Questions like this raise serious concerns about user privacy and rights. While the healthcare industry is highly regulated, questions arise on the regulations of these applications, which may not fall under the well-established industry and healthcare domain regulations and hence the app developers may not be obligated to adhere to the data handling practices.

Under the hood of the AI applications and systems making the predictions are the machine learning models which are trained on vast amounts of data. While these early detections and predictions are a huge advantage, it also raises some questions about the predictions. For example, if the model used in a healthcare system is trained on the data points from the population in one part of the world, would it be able to predict on the unseen patient data from another part of the world? So, can healthcare products, with AI embedded, which are highly accurate in one continent be equally accurate in another continent, or even another country differing in terms of language or cultural variations. Manifestation of many mental health conditions is highly influenced by cultural factors, thus there are chances of a particular application not yielding reliable prediction in other parts of the globe.

As the use of AI-driven systems increase in the healthcare domain, it is important for the doctors and healthcare professionals to not only understand the systems, and interpret the results correctly, but to understand the nuances of the systems so that they can understand limitations, spot any anomalies, and detect any potential errors or bias in the outcomes. In many cases, a deeper understanding of these nuances is necessary to communicate with patients and explain the basis of the decisions and potential risks.

Ethical Challenges in AI

In this section, we will explore the key ethical challenges in AI in greater detail. Ethical challenges in AI are a general issue across domains and industries. Specifically in the mental health domain, AI has many challenges, and it starts with the *data* that is used for training and building the models.

Data is the fundamental building block on which machine learning models are developed. However, having unbiased data may be a challenge. The training data may be biased and may not have an adequate representation of gender, age, race, ethnicity, regions of the world, etc. Hence a model trained on the data may not have a desired success level on underrepresented groups and may have a challenge for widespread use across different demography. There is also a need for user consent when an individual's health data is to be used for analysis and model development purposes, and common people may not be fully informed on how their health data be used. There are challenges to privacy and safety of health data, including the risk of cyber theft and data leakage, which may impact general people's right to privacy and dignity. There is stigma of individuals involved, and the leakage of these sensitive data may harm individuals.

As we delve deeper into each of the topics, it is important to remember that the goal of AI should be to augment human capabilities, not to replace them and such technological advancements are for the benefit of society at large, and reflect the human values like fairness, respect, responsibility, inclusiveness, and diversity.

Algorithmic Bias

Bias is a disproportionate weight in favour of or against an idea or thing, usually in a way that is inaccurate, closed-minded, prejudicial, or unfair (Wikipedia, n.d.). Some may tend to believe that humans have bias, but machines cannot be biased. However, in AI and machine learning that can be the farthest from the truth. Bias, or algorithmic bias, as is more specifically called in programming and machine learning terminology, is one of the biggest challenges of machine learning, and can be induced through data or decisions made by people.

In the healthcare domain, AI systems may help automate diagnosis and treatment and reduce cognitive biases in the decision-making of healthcare professionals. However, the AI systems themselves may inherently be biased in the way they have been developed, and due to the biased data on which the models have been trained on. As an example, a machine learning model trained on a dataset of people from the western part of the world to detect a disease, may not be as accurate to detect the disease in people from the eastern part of the world. Bias may be built into the system in the way decisions were taken to collect the data, to build the model, and in various stages of the development process. Due to the reach of digital technology, data across all demography may not even be available. The poorer communities may not have access to digital technologies and possibly the data from those communities were never collected. These societal reasons are the reasons for inherent bias in many datasets.

Let us consider an example of the usage of facial recognition software in computer vision which is increasingly being used in surveillance systems, airport and border control, and various biometric facial applications. These systems impact people's lives and are expected to be accurate. If these systems make a mistake, it can create a significant impact on individual's lives, for example a security surveillance system wrongly identifying the face of an innocent citizen as of a criminal. In the research paper *Gender Shades: Intersectional Accuracy Disparities in Commercial Gender Classification* (Buolamwini & Gebru, 2018) evaluated proprietary facial analysis services from three leading tech companies. The services used for gender classification were found to be discriminating based on classes like race and gender. Some of the key findings from the study depicted that the classifiers performed better on male faces than on female faces and performed better on lighter skin tone faces than on darker faces. The worst performance was observed to be on darker female faces. Proprietary software may not always disclose the underlying detail on how the models were trained and how the performance benchmarks were observed in testing, so the reason for the bias may not be known to the public, however issues like these are a cause of major concern. In earlier chapters, we discussed how facial expressions can be used for early identification for relapse prevention. In event such facial recognition software's embedded with a mental health application are biased for individuals of particular age group, sex or any other socio-demographic information, the prediction value as well as further consequences for the individual could be very distressing.

The companies building the software have the responsibility to address issues like these to prevent any discrimination and impact when used in real-world situations (Fig. 12.3).

Bias can exist at all stages in the life cycle of machine learning projects. Any machine learning project starts with the data. There can be societal bias reflected in the datasets with the data itself being biased due to social reasons. For example, a recruitment dataset built to screen suitable candidates for technology roles may give preferences to male candidates, if there is not enough representation of women in the original dataset. This could arise because of a lesser percentage of women who are in the tech industry compared to women. When a sample of data is chosen from the larger population, the sample may not be a true representation of the population. Also, even when the sample is a true representation of the population, there could be imbalances in the data, for example exceedingly small percentages of patients may be diagnosed with a disease in the complete dataset. In cases like these, model accuracy can also not be the measurement parameter to judge the performance of the system. For example, a dataset may have 0.15% of patients who are impacted by depression and 99.85% who are not. So even if the model predicts all patients as healthy and not be able to detect depression at all, it will still have an accuracy of 99.85. These are the kind of issues that need to be addressed in the design and development phase, by choosing the appropriate metrics for measurement. The training data also must

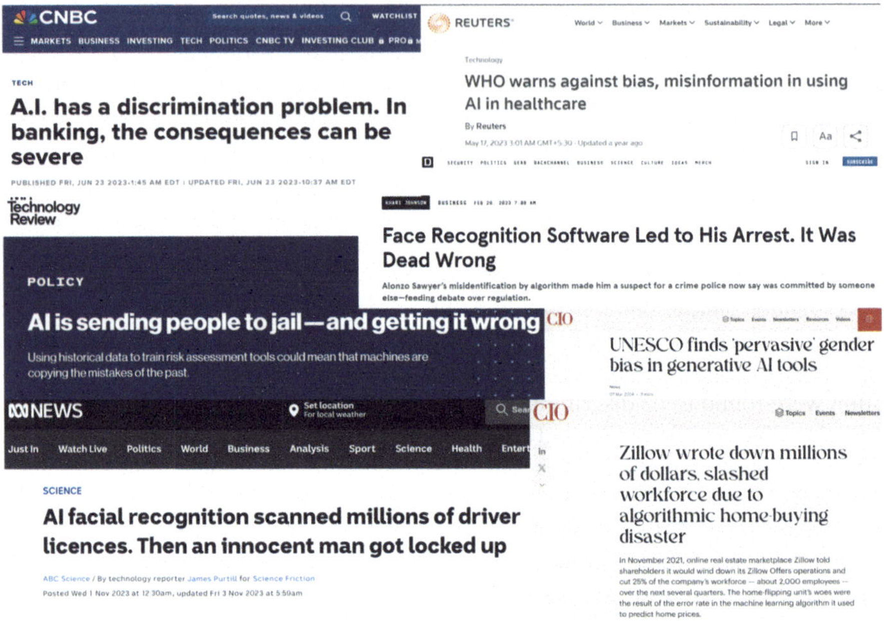

Fig. 12.3 Screenshots from News headlines on AI bias impacting human lives (CNBC, 2023; Hao, 2019, 2020; Olavsrud, 2024; Purtill, 2023; Reuters, 2023; Tucci, 2023)

have a fair representation of the population where the system will be used. A face recognition system developed with data from the western part of the world may not accurately identify the gender of people from the eastern part of the world.

The development and training phase may get induced with human biases. For example, a dataset may be prepared by imputing certain missing values based on human decision-making and these human decisions may lead to bias in the datasets. The choice of evaluation metrics may influence the way the model's performance is understood. Human interpretation of results from the AI systems may be biased. Developers should focus on the techniques available to identify these biases and mitigate them at each stage of the process. Bias is a major cause of concern and is an active field of research to improve the fairness of the systems for the larger good of society.

AI systems are often believed to be biased due to technical reasons; however, the bias often originates due to human, systemic and institutional reasons. National Institute of Standards and Technology (NIST) in its publication *Towards a Standard for Identifying and Managing Bias in Artificial Intelligence* (Schwartz et al., 2022) recommends not only to look at the data used to train the models and the machine learning process, but to also review the societal factors that influence how the AI systems are developed. This comprehensive approach is necessary to ensure that bias in AI systems is mitigated, and trust is increased for the users of the systems.

Transparency

As more decisions are driven by AI applications which are impacting human lives, the need for transparency is increasing. For example, when a loan gets rejected by a bank, or a job applicant's resume does not get selected for an interview, or a facial recognition or surveillance system flags an individual as an offender, a natural question that arises for the impacted person is, *why* did that happen? Why was the loan application rejected? Why did the person not get selected? Why did the facial recognition system flag the person as an offender?

This leads to the need for transparency in AI systems. The impacted persons have a right to know why the decision was taken. The authorities also need to be able to justify why the decision was made and explain it to the impacted person and often to society at large. There are situations when decisions may lead to litigations and in the court of law the justifications become the crucial point of contention. When there are consequences of the decisions, it is also a moral obligation of the authorities to explain to the impacted person why the decision was taken. Stating that the AI system took the decision is not a good enough justification.

Transparency is contextual, and appropriate levels of transparency may be required depending on the situation in which it is discussed and may vary based on the stakeholders. The right balance is necessary between transparency and secrecy. Depending on the context, a system may need to have varying amounts of transparency for different stakeholders. For example, a mental health app sensing suicidal thoughts in its user would alert the treating therapist, but not necessarily a distant contact. While there is a need for transparency in AI systems, there is a need to have contextual balance between transparency and secrecy.

Privacy and Security

The first step to data collection from a privacy aspect is to take *consent* from the users, clarifying clearly why the data will be collected, what will be the purpose in which the data will be used, how the data will be anonymized, and which parties will have access to the data. This is incredibly difficult and complex though in the real world. The data collected may be used for specific purposes at the time of collection, however in future that data may be used for some other purposes as well. At the time of taking the consent the future usage of the data may not even be clearly known, particularly as vast amounts of data points get correlated to solve various use cases.

To protect the privacy of individuals it is crucial to maintain the security of the data to ensure there are no data breaches by bad actors. In a connected world, cyber-attacks, including ransomware attacks, have become common. Organizations and individuals dealing with sensitive data must have security mechanisms in place to protect from threats and cyber-attacks. The data collected also needs to be anonymized to prevent any leakage of personal identifiable information to unauthorized persons.

Copyright and Intellectual Property

Generative AI and the Large Language Models have raised concerns about copyright issues, and there are several lawsuits that have been filed by content owners against the large tech companies developing these models. The Large Language Models are trained on a huge corpus of text, images, and videos available publicly and the companies developing the models may not have had the permission to use them. There are concerns of writers and artists that their literary work, images, and work of art have been used by the companies to train the models and no attribution has been provided to the original content creators.

These are complex issues, and the regulatory and legal framework are currently evolving around the AI ecosystem. Guidelines are being formulated for copyrights and intellectual property rights for the usage of data for model training and the content that is AI generated. As the regulatory and legal positions around Generative AI evolve, there is a cautious approach being taken by organizations for adopting Generative AI tools in their business to avoid any legal and reputational impact.

Accountability

While the possibility remains that an AI system may make a wrong decision and cause harm, the system cannot be held liable for mistakes or malfunctioning. The organizations designing and developing the systems need to be responsible and accountable for any impact caused by these systems. However, in real-world situations the demarcation of accountability and responsibility may not be straightforward to define. We are aware of the accident that happened in the United States in 2019, in which two people were hit by a self-driving car and died. The man in the vehicle was charged with criminal prosecution (Feingold, 2022). So, what happens if an individual diagnosed with a mental ill health condition using a mental health chatbot or other application commits suicide. These are complex cases, and contextual evaluations need to be done including technological failures and human negligence.

Using AI for decision-making comes with its own risks, often with a lack of control by humans. However, the organizations and individuals building the AI systems should still be held accountable for any adverse effect that may happen due to the outcome of AI systems. To manage these complexities and mitigate the challenges, AI governance plays a vital role to ensure AI is being used in a responsible, secure, and ethical manner and the AI systems are trustworthy.

Trustworthy AI Systems

The National Institute of Standard and Technology (NIST) released Artificial Intelligence Risk Management Framework (AI RMF 1.0) to provide organizations and individuals with approaches that would increase the trustworthiness of the AI Systems, when adopted in their end-to-end lifecycle. The framework is an excellent resource to consider for responsible design, development, deployment, and use of AI systems. This helps to have a structured approach towards managing risks for AI systems and applications.

According to the framework, there are key characteristics that can increase the trustworthiness of the AI systems (Tabassi, 2023) (Fig. 12.4).

Valid & Reliable: It is necessary for the AI systems to produce valid and reliable outputs, for it to be trustworthy and hence is depicted as the foundation block applicable for each of the other characteristics. An AI system is valid means that the system meets the requirements for its intended use, and being reliable ensures that the system performs without failure. This is related to the *accuracy* and *robustness* of the machine learning models to maintain their performance under a variety of circumstances. The AI systems should be designed to minimize potential negative impacts and include human intervention where the AI systems cannot detect and correct the errors. For example, a mental health app upon sensing self-harming ideas in the user must alert the approved and consented therapist and or family members.

Accountable and Transparent: The vertical block represents that it relates to all the other trustworthy characteristics. The builders and developers of the AI systems should be accountable for the output of the systems they build and maintain. For the systems to be trustworthy it is necessary for the systems to be transparent in the way it is designed and deployed. Depending on the role of the stakeholders, the more understandable the system is, there will be more confidence in the output generated by these systems, effectively increasing the trust in the system. Transparency and understanding of the inner working of the system also lead to taking conscious corrective measures when the outputs are not in line with expectations.

Safe: Safety of the AI systems is of paramount importance. As domains like self-driving cars and health care are having AI embedded in the systems, it is crucial to ensure that the systems are not imposing any risk to human life, health, property, and

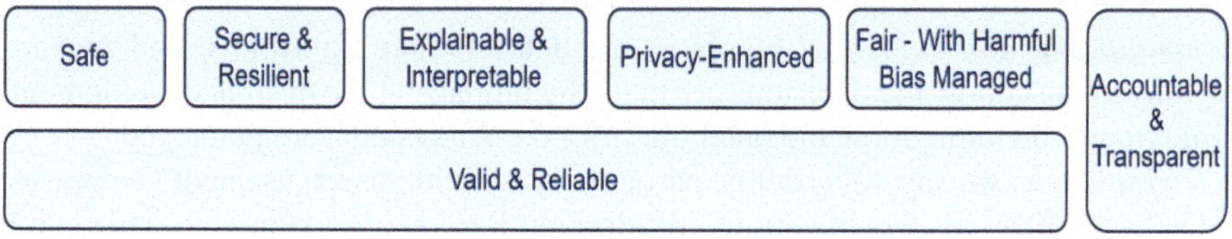

Fig. 12.4 Characteristics of trustworthy AI systems published by NIST

its operating environment. At every stage of the AI lifecycle, from design, development, and deployment, it is important to build in safety measures and perform rigorous testing, real-time monitoring, and take actions to mitigate any risks that may arise in practice. The safety measures should also consider the safety standards of the respective industries to be built in and addressed within the AI systems. In terms of mental health, all recommendations or suggestions from AI-based apps or avatars should be based on evidence-based scientific medical literature.

Secure and Resilient: AI systems need to have guardrails to ensure that the confidentiality, integrity, and availability of the systems are maintained under all circumstances. The systems should be secured to prevent, defend against, respond to, and recover from adversarial situations. The systems should be resilient to restore normal operations after any negative event. The data, models, and the overall systems should have security and resiliency built in to protect against any unforeseen events and bad actors. For the consumers of the systems, this is extremely crucial to ensure privacy and security of their personal information. Mental ill health in itself carries big stigma, and breach of sensitive patient data may have a major detrimental impact on the patients if exposed to unauthorized personnel.

Explainable and Interpretable: Explainability refers to understanding the functionality of the models and the systems. The developers of the AI systems should be able to understand the functionality of each component of the system, which would enable better documentation, troubleshooting and fixing any bugs in the system. This would build confidence in how the systems work and not just treat the machine learning models and the neural networks as a black box. Interpretability is about comprehending the output in the context of the system's intended function. Explainability is understanding *how* the system made the decision, and interpretability is understanding *why* the system made the decision. Having a complete understanding of this is important to have control on the functioning of the systems, mitigate any risks and thus build trust in the ability of the systems.

Privacy-Enhanced: Privacy is required to ensure people's personal details, information and identities are protected. There is a lot of sensitive data that is handled by AI systems and appropriate security guardrails need to be put in place to safeguard from any data breaches.

Fair with Harmful Bias Managed: Fairness in AI means that the models do not discriminate one group over another. In the lifecycle of an AI system, there could be *systemic* bias in the complete lifecycle of the AI system based on the environment, *computational and statistical* biases in the datasets and algorithms, and *human-cognitive* bias in how the decisions are made by humans in the design, development, deployment, including how the outcome from the AI systems are perceived.

To build trustworthy AI systems, particularly with increased usage of Generative AI in the applications, organizations are adopting *Responsible AI* practices to govern the lifecycle of the AI systems to minimize risk and negative impacts.

Responsible AI

In the end-to-end lifecycle of an AI application, from design and development to deployment, usage, and maintenance, decisions made at each stage significantly impact the outcomes. Organizations working on AI are establishing Responsible AI principles and practices to navigate this journey, ensuring that the outcomes from AI systems are trustworthy and instil confidence in the users. AI is developing at a rapid pace and is being utilized across various domains and use cases, including those with significant human impact, such as medical diagnosis and further management. However, it is clear from some real-world cases that AI can still make mistakes in its outcomes.

In 2018 it was reported (Dastin, 2018) that Amazon was experimenting with a hiring tool using AI to filter the top resumes of candidates. However, Amazon realized that the tool was discriminating against female candidates in its filtering process and scrapped the tool. AI systems may encounter and emphasize the need to understand how the algorithms make the decisions. The data on which the model was trained on was from the past 10 years and had more resumes from men due to the presence of a higher percentage of men in the tech industry compared to women. So, the model preferred male candidates and downgraded resumes where it found the word *women,* like *women's chess club captain.* It downgraded the resumes of candidates from all-women's colleges. This case brings out the limitations of the AI systems, and depicts the importance of understanding the *training data,* and the social *bias* that may be ingrained in the datasets. For mental health-based applications, it can transpire in misidentifying individuals at risk or highly likely to have diagnosis of a certain disorder, because of their age, sex or other socio-demographic character.

In 2016 Microsoft launched Tay, an AI chatbot *"to experiment with and conduct research on conversational understanding"* (Leetaru, 2016). Tay was designed to learn over time from the conversational streams on Twitter. Unfortunately, Tay learnt toxicity from the Twitter data stream and started spitting out toxic responses, in absence of any content filter in the system. Microsoft had to discontinue Tay immediately due to the issues it faced in the real world. This instance makes it clear that the challenges encountered in real-world deployment can significantly differ from those expected during the development stage. So we need to mitigate the risk of use of toxic language by chatbots in the process of guiding individuals.

In real-world scenarios, it is often difficult to pre-empt what may go wrong. In the cases mentioned above, the leading companies that develop AI with the best of governance embedded in its processes and rich pool of expert talent, still face these challenges and there are unforeseen situations in which things go wrong. This necessitates a need to always be vigilant of potential issues and manage or mitigate these risks as much as possible.

The aim of Responsible AI practices is to identify potential issues and deliberate on the consequences at each stage of the AI lifecycle, recognize the limitations, and make informed decisions to mitigate the possibilities of harmful and negative impact on users and society. In absence of any universally accepted methodology or framework for Responsible AI, most organizations are setting their own Responsible AI principles and practices based on their organizational objectives and values, mostly incorporating a set of principles, such as fairness, transparency, privacy, and security.

While AI systems make decisions when implemented, it is humans who decide how to build these systems and let the AI generate the outcomes. For example, it is a human decision on which dataset to train the machine learning models, how that data is collected, what is included in the data sample, which algorithms to use, how to manage bias in the system and data, and even how to interpret the results. At every stage of the design and development process, it is the developers who make the decisions. Decisions need to be taken by humans on the trade-offs between several factors of performance and reliability in the design and development phase. Therefore, the guidelines and principles of Responsible AI play a significant role in ensuring that the decisions are made responsibly to avoid any negative consequences when the products are used in the real-world.

People make decisions based on their culture and values, which also leads to societal bias which gets infiltrated into the data that gets generated. These human decisions may reflect the way the AI systems are built, the way the datasets are generated, and may reflect in outcomes from the systems. When these decisions are made, it is also important to consider whether they are made ethically and societal aspects, like inclusiveness, accessibility, diversity, are considered and respected.

The use of Generative AI in applications has increased the complexity of the challenges even more. A key aspect of Responsible AI is ensuring fairness and mitigating potential biases. This is particularly relevant when considering the risks and challenges associated with Large Language Models (LLMs), which are trained on large corpus of data from the public internet. The use of Large Language Models has brought in other challenges like toxicity, hallucinations, and intellectual property issues.

Based on the datasets that the Large Language Models are trained on, they can generate *toxic content*, which can be harmful and discriminatory towards certain groups. To address this issue, it is important to filter the training data to ensure that toxic contents are not being fed into the LLMs for training and content-filters are used appropriately in the systems. The LLMs pose another challenge in *hallucinating*, generating content that is not true, incorrect, and even unreal. When the LLMs do not find an appropriate response based on the corpus it was trained on, they start generating content which may be baseless. This is a serious challenge as the generated content may likely sound so true. To mitigate this issue, LLMs are often augmented with verified external sources to validate and cite the response before it is presented to the user. Another issue that has caused several lawsuits against companies developing LLMs is intellectual property rights. There are many cases of intellectual property rights issues that have been raised due to models generating content that infringes copyright laws.

Organizations are taking active steps to address these issues, through Responsible AI principles and practices, and AI governance and accountability is being exercised through the lifecycle of AI projects. There are steps being taken globally to establish governance framework for usage of AI.

The European Union AI Act

In March 2024, the European Union Parliament approved the Artificial Intelligence Act (AI Act), which is considered as the first comprehensive legal framework for governing AI systems (McCallum et al., n.d.). The Act defines the requirements for AI systems that would mitigate AI risks and is designed with a goal to make AI human centric. The Act has a global significance as this is applicable to all companies developing and deploying AI systems in the European Union, irrespective of where the companies are located, and in which country the AI systems are developed.

It provides a guideline for AI developers and deployers regarding the uses of AI to protect the safety and fundamental rights of people and businesses (European Commission, n.d.). It defines a risk-based framework where each AI system would fall into either of the categories. It would be necessary for the AI systems to undergo an assessment, comply with the requirements defined in the Act before they can be released in the market for use. The framework defines four levels of risk for the AI systems (Fig. 12.5).

Unacceptable risk: All the AI systems that impact the safety, livelihood, and rights of people will be banned.

High risk: These systems need to strictly pass an assessment before they can be put on the market for general use. These apps must adhere to a set of obligations like usage of high-quality datasets to minimize bias and discriminatory outcomes,

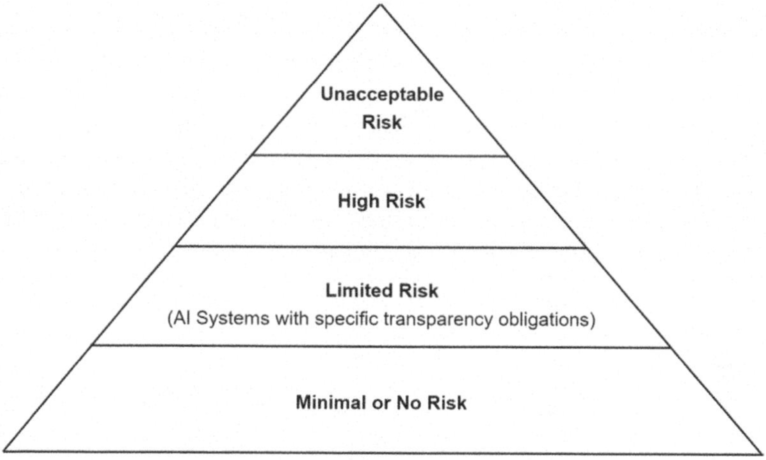

Fig. 12.5 Four levels of risk for AI Systems

and must be robust, secure and accurate. All activities in the app must be logged for traceability and detailed documentation must be made available for deployers and authorities for assessment. Adequate measures must be taken into consideration for risk assessment and mitigation and appropriate human oversight would be required to minimize any risk. Some of the AI Systems identified as high risk are systems that put the health and safety of the public at risk, like transportation systems. AI systems impacting the lives of people like systems used for selection of students in educational courses, selection of candidates for employment, border control systems, judicial systems, and safety components of products like the technology used in robotic surgery fall in this risk category.

Limited risk: This category specifically calls out the AI apps where more transparency is required. For example, AI chatbots should make it clear to the public that the conversation is happening with an AI agent. AI-generated content must be identifiable as AI generated, and text generated by AI on matters of public interest must be labelled as AI generated.

Minimal or no risk: Minimal risk AI systems, for example AI-enabled video games, spam filters, etc. can be used freely. Most AI apps in the market fall in this category.

All these measures and establishment of guidelines and frameworks would help in increasing the trust of people in AI systems, minimize the risk and prevent the systems from being misused and harm segments of society. The focus is on human-centric AI which respects human dignity and increases trust in the systems while fostering technological innovation and advancement.

Conclusion

As the scope and implication of AI broadens with each passing day, the need for ethical practice of AI-based application in health and mental health in particular also gets a boost. The AI-based applications bring promising and novel approaches to increase efficacy in mental health care, the concerns regarding data safety, accuracy of data analysis, and bias need to be addressed by developers. The applications need to be transparent yet secure and capable enough to filter unwanted learning from the dataset. There is a need for uniform regulations on the development and accountability of the AI-based mental healthcare applications.

References

Buolamwini, J., & Gebru, T. (2018). Gender shades: Intersectional accuracy disparities in commercial gender classification. In S. A. Friedler & C. Wilson (Eds.), *Proceedings of Machine Learning Research* (p. 81). PMLR.

CNBC. (2023, June 23). A.I. has a discrimination problem. In *Banking, the consequences can be severe*. CNBC. https://www.cnbc.com/2023/06/23/ai-has-a-discrimination-problem-in-banking-that-can-be-devastating.html

Dastin, J. (2018, October 11). *Insight: Amazon scraps secret AI recruiting tool that showed bias against women*. Reuters. https://www.reuters.com/article/amazon-com-jobs-automation/insight-amazon-scraps-secret-ai-recruiting-tool-that-showed-bias-against-women-idINKCN1MK0AH/?edition-redirect=in

European Commission. (n.d.). *AI act*. Shaping Europe's Digital Future. Retrieved April 16, 2024, from https://digital-strategy.ec.europa.eu/en/policies/regulatory-framework-ai

Feingold, S. (2022, August 25). *Who is to blame if a self-driving car crashes?* World Economic Forum. https://www.weforum.org/agenda/2022/08/who-is-to-blame-if-a-self-driving-car-crashes/

Hao, K. (2019, January 21). AI is sending people to jail—And getting it wrong. *MIT Technology Review*. https://www.technologyreview.com/2019/01/21/137783/algorithms-criminal-justice-ai/

Hao, K. (2020, June 24). *A face recognition company wrongly identified a man as a criminal. It was dead wrong*. Wired. https://www.wired.com/story/face-recognition-software-led-to-his-arrest-it-was-dead-wrong/

Leetaru, K. (2016, March 24). How Twitter corrupted Microsoft's Tay: A crash course in the dangers of AI in the real world. *Forbes*. https://www.forbes.com/sites/kalevleetaru/2016/03/24/how-twitter-corrupted-microsofts-tay-a-crash-course-in-the-dangers-of-ai-in-the-real-world/?sh=62ca862126d2

McCallum, S., McMahon, L., & Singleton, T. (n.d.). *MEPs approve world's first comprehensive AI law*. BBC.com. Retrieved April 16, 2024, from https://www.bbc.com/news/technology-68546450

Olavsrud, T. (2024, October 2). *12 famous AI disasters*. CIO. https://www.cio.com/article/190888/5-famous-analytics-and-ai-disasters.html

Purtill, J. (2023, November 1). AI facial recognition scanned millions of driver licences. Then an innocent man got locked up. *ABC News*. https://www.abc.net.au/news/science/2023-11-01/ai-facial-recognition-robert-williams-crime-prison/103032148

Reuters. (2023, May 16). *WHO warns against bias, misinformation in using AI in healthcare*. Reuters. https://www.reuters.com/technology/who-warns-against-bias-misinformation-using-ai-healthcare-2023-05-16/

Schwartz, R., Vassilev, A., Greene, K., Perine, L., Burt, A., & Hall, P. (2022). *Towards a standard for identifying and managing bias in Artificial Intelligence*. https://doi.org/10.6028/NIST.SP.1270

Tabassi, E. (2023). *Artificial intelligence risk management framework (AI RMF 1.0)*. https://doi.org/10.6028/NIST.AI.100-1

Tucci, L. (2023, October 23). *UNESCO finds pervasive gender bias in generative AI tools*. CIO. https://www.cio.com/article/1312311/unesco-finds-pervasive-gender-bias-in-generative-ai-tools.html

Wikipedia. (n.d.). *Bias*. Wikipedia. Retrieved April 11, 2024, from https://en.wikipedia.org/wiki/Bias

Chapter 13
AI Vision for Mental Health in 2025 and Beyond

Abstract In this final chapter, we will share our take on the future possibilities of AI in mental health care. Emerging AI technologies, including advancements in Generative AI and natural language processing, promise to further integrate AI into diagnosing, treating, and preventing mental health problems beyond what we have discussed so far in previous chapters. The chapter provides insight into mental health domains where AI can bring impactful change in coming years and need focus.

Keywords Emerging AI technologies · Personalization · Global accessibility · Human expertise

The Key Areas

AI is going to shift from a supporting tool to a critical collaborator in full mental health ecosystems, incorporating wearables, predictive analytics, and personalised care tactics. In this developing paradigm, artificial intelligence will use data from smartphones and wearable devices such as smartwatches and fitness trackers to deliver real-time insights into a person's mental state. The key domains where AI is poised for advancement are:

- Neurotechnology
- Genetic therapy
- Focus on Personalization
- Community-based treatment
- Global accessibility
- Collaboration among stakeholders
- Balancing AI and human expertise

Neurotechnology: Neurotechnology which mainly understands brain functions and its process is used in a variety of disciplines, including health, medical treatment, education, workplace management, and sports is going to be a major impact. However, its key applications including brain imaging, neurostimulation,

S. Halder et al., *Navigating AI in Mental Health Care*,
https://doi.org/10.1007/978-981-96-9744-1_13

and neurodevices are still used in very limited way. Brain imaging, such as MRI, maps brain activity and is used to diagnose illnesses including tumours and strokes while also providing information about brain function. Neurostimulation techniques such as Transcranial Magnetic Stimulation (TMS), Transcranial Direct Current Stimulation (tDCS), and low-field magnetic stimulation alter brain activity and are used to treat spinal cord and nerve disorders. Neurodevices, which include neural implants, offer promise in treating neurological illnesses such as Parkinson's disease, albeit they are still in the research stage. These innovations have enormous potential to improve health care and overall well-being. In the future, improved brain-computer interfaces (BCIs) and robotics are projected to have a transformational role in treating refractory illnesses such as chronic schizophrenia or irreversible condition like dementia. These AI-powered devices can interpret brain data and identify patterns that correspond to symptoms like hallucinations and delusions. Real-time brain monitoring allows patients to receive biofeedback to help them regulate their emotional states. AI-powered cognitive rehabilitation programmes can improve attention and memory through targeted neurofeedback, and predictive analytics allows for exact prescription planning by analysing individual neural responses, minimizing reliance on trial-and-error procedures. Robotics combined with BCIs can provide critical support for daily activities like as mobility and self-care, enabling greater autonomy and increasing the quality of life for people with chronic schizophrenia or dementia.

Genetic therapy Is another domain which has a great role to play in future mental health treatment. AI is revolutionizing gene therapy by improving the development, optimization, and implementation of treatments. It aids in designing synthetic DNA sequences that can precisely regulate gene expression in specific cells, which could lead to targeted therapies for conditions such as Parkinson's, metabolic disorders, and blood diseases. Genetic data can reveal predispositions to certain mental health conditions, while behavioural patterns, such as daily routines or stress triggers can help in planning patterns. AI plays a crucial role in identifying individuals at higher risk of genetic disorders by analysing vast genetic databases, enabling early detection and intervention. Additionally, AI enhances patient care by predicting how individuals will respond to gene therapies, allowing for personalized treatment plans. In the realm of gene editing, AI aids in the design of guide RNAs that assure high editing accuracy while minimizing off-target effects, boosting intervention efficiency and safety. Furthermore, AI can model intricate biological processes involved in gene delivery, such as the behaviour of vectors and peptides in creating holes, allowing for the refinement of delivery systems. Overall, artificial intelligence is changing gene therapy by making it more precise, efficient, and personalized.

Focus of Personalization: The expanding use of personalized digital technology in mental health treatment has the potential to completely transform how mental health is monitored, diagnosed, and treated. We already have powerful smart gadgets measuring physical metrics like step count, calorie intake, heart rate, and body mass index, but the same level of complexity is increasingly required in the arena of mental health. Smartphones and smartwatches with built-in sensors can be used for real-time behavioural tracking, including mood, stress levels, and emotional tension. This is going to prepare the way for a new era of mental health care in which the emphasis switches from reactive to proactive measures, aided by real-time insights into the user's psychological condition.

Artificial intelligence (AI) is transitioning from a support tool to a key player in this ecosystem, providing predictive analytics and personalized treatment solutions. Wearable gadgets, such as fitness trackers and smartwatches, are expected to play an important role in collecting physiological data, such as heart rate variability, sleep patterns, and physical activity levels. These markers provide essential information for AI systems to identify early signs of stress, anxiety, or depression. By continuously analysing these inputs, AI can detect possible mental health crises before they occur, allowing for timely interventions to avert escalation. For example, a sudden rise in heart rate variability mixed with interrupted sleep patterns may indicate heightened stress, prompting the system to recommend relaxation activities or perhaps notify a healthcare physician for additional action.

Incorporating personalized care strategies enhances the efficiency of these improvements. AI systems may adjust therapy recommendations to an individual's specific genetic, behavioural, and environmental characteristics, ensuring that interventions are appropriate for their circumstances and preferences. Unlike generalized treatment regimens, this technique ensures a more targeted, successful therapy regimen that is meaningful to the patient. For example, someone with a history of anxiety and low social support may be given digital therapy content aimed at improving emotional resilience, whereas another person with identical symptoms but different environmental triggers may be given a mindfulness-based intervention. One of the most intriguing characteristics of these kinds of devices is their capacity to detect minor changes in psychological states. Beyond typical mental health indicators, these systems aim to monitor finer cognitive skills such as memory, decision-making, adaptability, and planning on an ongoing basis. Current cognitive apps appear simple and may lack the precision required for effective mental health interventions. To overcome this gap, sophisticated technologies are required that focus on high-resolution monitoring of cognitive processes and provide practical recommendations for improvement. AI-powered mental health technologies will also solve precision issues by incorporating continuous feedback loops. For example, if a user exhibits indicators of cognitive decline or impaired decision-making, the device may provide specific cognitive training exercises or initiate early clinical assessments.

This continual connection between the user and the technology ensures that even modest changes in mental and cognitive health are identified, allowing for rapid adjustments to treatment strategies. In this changing paradigm, digital mental health technology will no longer be passive tools, but rather active participants in improving mental well-being. This ecosystem, which combines wearable technology, advanced AI analytics, and personalized therapies, has the potential to transform mental health care by making it more accessible, responsive, and suited to individual requirements. As these technologies mature, they have the potential to alter how mental health is understood and treated, resulting in more effective outcomes.

Community-Based Treatment: One of the major reasons, why mental health is not accessible to all is lack of required trained professionals, stigma as well cost to certain extent. Trained professionals are mostly concentrated in big cities and metros which are often not cost effective for all. On the contrary the low-cost public services are too crowded impacting services delivery. Primary prevention strategies though are effective do lack mass level implementation. Thus, this is one domain where AI can have large impact. There is a dire need of shifting from clinic-based treatment to community to enhance reachability, availability and affordability of mental health services.

As digital technology grows more prevalent in society, tasks and services that were formerly handled manually and often slowly are now completed more efficiently via automated technological systems. However, while many businesses have embraced new technologies to improve efficiency and responsiveness, mental health care has not made the same progress. Mental health care is unavailable, complicated to navigate, reactive, and slow to deliver, leaving mental health consumers frustrated and carers burnt out. People now have more access to information, including medical information and personal health data, than ever before. In today's landscape, when "on-demand" services are becoming more common, mental health customers and MHPs may expect similar responsiveness. As a result, many people are turning to digital products and services that are designed to meet their urgent requirements. Young people, for example, are open and enthusiastic in adopting a variety of digital technology to promote mental health, and many physicians are already using these tools into normal therapy.

The shift from traditional clinic-based mental health treatment to community-based care, aided by digital technologies, is an important step towards resolving challenges of accessibility, availability, and affordability. Clinic-based services frequently require consumers to travel, adhere to stringent appointment schedules, and pay hefty fees, making them inaccessible to many people, particularly those in rural or underdeveloped areas. Community-based digital solutions, on the other hand, can help to close the gap by providing flexible, on-demand access to mental health support. Mobile applications, teletherapy platforms, and online support groups enable people to get care from the comfort of their own homes, dramatically increasing reachability by breaking down geographical obstacles.

Digital technologies boost availability by providing scalable solutions that can serve a larger population at the same time. Automated mental health applications, chatbots, and AI-powered interventions can give early support to users, decreasing the workload on mental health professionals (MHPs) and ensuring that people in need receive prompt assistance. This model not only optimizes the use of limited resources, but it also ensures that individuals can receive care without having to wait weeks or months, as is common in clinic-based settings.

Another significant benefit of community-based digital mental health care is its low cost. Traditional services are frequently expensive due to the overhead costs connected with operating physical facilities and recruiting full-time employees. In contrast, digital solutions lower these costs by employing automation, internet infrastructure, and scalable technology, making mental health care cheaper for both providers and patients. Community-based digital interventions can provide tiered models of care, with basic services free or low-cost and highly personalized interventions offered at a premium, providing inclusion across income strata. By adopting this paradigm, mental health treatments can become more accessible, efficient, and egalitarian, ultimately serving and benefiting a broader population.

Most importantly the technological advances can be used by both public and private players.

Global accessibility: AI holds the potential to democratize mental health care, addressing disparities in access for underserved populations worldwide. Mobile apps and AI-driven chatbots are key tools in this transformation, offering affordable, scalable, and 24/7 support to individuals in remote or resource-limited areas. These tools can provide basic therapeutic interventions, educational resources, and crisis support, making mental health care more accessible than ever before. In addition to their cost-effectiveness, AI solutions overcome language barriers through natural language processing and multilingual capabilities, ensuring that help is available in the user's preferred language. AI-powered platforms can also adapt to cultural sensitivities, delivering context-appropriate care that resonates with diverse populations. Moreover, these tools enable individuals to seek help anonymously, which can be particularly beneficial in communities where mental health stigma is prevalent. By breaking down geographical, financial, and cultural barriers, AI is poised to transform mental health care into a universally accessible service, fostering equity and inclusion in global mental health initiatives.

Collaboration Among Stakeholders: Collaboration among AI experts, mental health providers, and policymakers is critical to the successful integration of artificial intelligence in mental health care. However, considerable issues can be developed as a result of these stakeholders' varying terminology, priorities, and views. Mental health experts have to prioritize clinical accuracy, patient safety, and ethical considerations while developing AI-powered solutions will ensure that they meet established healthcare standards and address patients' well-being. In contrast, AI professionals have to give importance technological feasibility, algorithm performance, and data utilization in order to create new and efficient solutions. Meanwhile, business developers are motivated by market demands, scalability, and profitability, seeking long-term and economically viable solutions. These contrasting priorities might lead to misunderstandings and delay efficient collaboration. To overcome these problems, it is critical to establish a shared language and goals. Regular interdisciplinary meetings and collaborative workshops can serve as a forum for open communication, allowing stakeholders to align their expectations and add their specific skills to the development process. Such initiatives can promote mutual understanding, knowledge exchange, and ensure that AI solutions are technically solid and clinically relevant.

Furthermore, policymakers play an important role in developing rules that strike a balance between innovation and ethical considerations, ensuring that AI-powered mental health solutions meet legal and ethical requirements. Stakeholders can collaborate to build artificial intelligence (AI) tools that are safe, effective, and easily accessible, ultimately enhancing mental health care outcomes and meeting the field's increasing need for digital solutions.

Balancing AI and Human Expertise: Just as scepticism has surrounded the use of AI in applications like self-driving cars, the integration of AI in mental health care is not without its challenges. Concerns around accuracy, reliability, and ethical implications raise legitimate questions about how these tools should be used. Mental health is deeply personal, and there is a critical need to ensure that AI systems operate responsibly and transparently. There are legitimate questions about whether AI can truly understand and address the complexities of human emotions and experiences. This scepticism emphasizes the importance of careful deployment, where AI is used as a complement rather than a replacement for human professionals. By involving experts in developing and overseeing these tools and maintaining strict ethical guidelines, the potential for harm can be minimized. While AI is poised to be a significant agent in accelerating and democratizing the mental health industry, the need for human expertise will remain essential and irreplaceable. Mental health, at its core, deals with deeply human emotional issues that require empathy, connection, and understanding. AI can analyse patterns, predict crises, and offer evidence-based recommendations, but it lacks the nuanced relational and emotional depth that a human therapist or mental health professional provides. The therapeutic alliance—the trust and bond between a client and a clinician—is a critical component of effective mental health care and cannot be replicated by technology.

Another crucial aspect of mental health is understanding the nature and origin of individuals' issues. This process often involves deep exploration, active listening, and a contextual understanding of personal experiences, all requiring human judgement and sensitivity. AI can assist in gathering data and providing insights, but humans must remain the final touchpoint in interpreting this information and implementing care. This collaborative relationship between AI and human professionals ensures that technology enhances, rather than replaces, mental health care's emotional and relational aspects. While AI is poised to be a significant agent in accelerating and democratizing the mental health industry, the need for human expertise will remain essential and irreplaceable. Mental health, at its core, deals with deeply human emotional issues that require empathy, connection, and understanding.

Conclusion: In coming years, AI will be a key player in services including mental health. The advancements in the domain have already shown the glimpses of its potentials, but it's overuse or unthoughtful and unethical use may have negative consequences. Many mental health issues stem from a lack of human connection and touchpoints, and an overreliance on AI might exacerbate these feelings of isolation. It is crucial to use AI as a supportive tool, not a replacement for human interaction. The balance between leveraging technological advancements and preserving the irreplaceable human elements of care will ensure that mental health services remain effective and compassionate.

Uncited References

Amazon AWS. (n.d.). *Building AI responsibly at AWS*. Amazon AWS. Retrieved April 9, 2024, from https://aws.amazon.com/machine-learning/responsible-ai/

American Psychiatric Association. (1994). *DSM-IV: Diagnostic and statistical manual of mental disorders* (4th ed.). American Psychiatric Association.

Batstra, L., Hadders-Algra, M., Nieweg, E., Van Tol, D., Pijl, S. J., & Frances, A. (2012). Childhood emotional and behavioral problems: Reducing overdiagnosis without risking undertreatment. *Developmental Medicine & Child Neurology, 54*(6), 492–494. https://doi.org/10.1111/j.1469-8749.2011.04176

Bearne, S. (n.d.). New AI systems collide with copyright law. *BBC News*. Retrieved April 17, 2024, from https://www.bbc.com/news/business-66231268

Chen, Z. S., Kulkarni, P. P., Galatzer-Levy, I. R., Bigio, B., Nasca, C., & Zhang, Y. (2022). Modern views of machine learning for precision psychiatry. *Patterns (New York, N.Y.), 3*(11), 100602. https://doi.org/10.1016/j.patter.2022.100602

Clementz, B. A., Sweeney, J. A., Hamm, J. P., Ivleva, E. I., Ethridge, L. E., Pearlson, G. D., Keshavan, M. S., & Tamminga, C. A. (2016). Identification of distinct psychosis biotypes using brain-based biomarkers. *The American Journal of Psychiatry, 173*(4), 373–384. https://doi.org/10.1176/appi.ajp.2015.14091200

Frances, A. (2013). The past, present and future of psychiatric diagnosis. *World Psychiatry: Official Journal of the World Psychiatric Association (WPA), 12*(2), 111–112. https://doi.org/10.1002/wps.20027

Google. (n.d.). *Responsible AI practices*. Google. Retrieved April 7, 2024, from https://ai.google/responsibility/responsible-ai-practices/

Hua, Y., Liu, F., Yang, K., Li, Z., Sheu, Y., Zhou, P., Moran, L. V., Ananiadou, S., & Beam, A. (2024). Large language models in mental health care: A scoping review. *Current Treatment Options in Psychiatry, 12*(1), 1–18.

Jiang, F., Jiang, Y., Zhi, H., Dong, Y., Li, H., Ma, S., Wang, Y., Dong, Q., Shen, H., & Wang, Y. (2017). Artificial intelligence in healthcare: Past, present, and future. *Stroke and Vascular Neurology, 2*(4), 230–243. https://doi.org/10.1136/svn-2017-000101

Luccioni, A. S., Viguier, S., & Ligozat, A. L. (2023). Estimating the carbon footprint of BLOOM, a 176B parameter language model. *Journal of Machine Learning Research, 24*, 1–15.

Menon, G. (n.d.). *Mental-health-mistral-7b-instructv0.2-finetuned-V2*. Hugging Face. Retrieved March 31, 2024, from https://huggingface.co/GRMenon/mental-health-mistral-7b-instructv0.2-finetuned-V2

Microsoft. (n.d.). *Microsoft AI - Responsible AI - Principles and approach*. Microsoft. Retrieved April 7, 2024, from https://www.microsoft.com/en-us/ai/principles-and-approach

Narayanan, K. (2021). *AI in medicine and healthcare—A brief history & implications for the future*. Analytics India Magazine. Retrieved December 5, 2023, from https://analyticsindiamag.com/ai-in-medicine-and-healthcare-a-brief-history-implications-for-the-future/

NIHR Evidence; Artificial intelligence: 10 promising interventions for healthcare; July 2023; https://doi.org/10.3310/nihrevidence_59502

Raghavan, P. (2024, February 23). Gemini image generation got it wrong. We'll do better. *Google Blog—The Keyword*. https://blog.google/products/gemini/gemini-image-generation-issue/

Taska, B., Samila, S., Azar, J., Giné, M., & Alekseeva, L. (2020, May 3). *The demand for AI skills in the labour market*. Centre for Economic Policy Research (CEPR). https://cepr.org/voxeu/columns/demand-ai-skills-labour-market

UCSF Department of Psychiatry and Behavioral Sciences. (n.d.). *Useful wellness and mental health apps. Mental health resources for crisis*. Retrieved March 30, 2024, from https://psychiatry.ucsf.edu/copingresources/apps

World Health Organization. (n.d.). *Mental disorders*. Retrieved January 25, 2024, from https://www.who.int/news-room/fact-sheets/detail/mental-disorders

Yang, K., Zhang, T., Kuang, Z., Xie, Q., Huang, J., & Ananiadou, S. (2023). *MentaLLaMA: Interpretable mental health analysis on social media with large language models*. https://doi.org/10.1145/3589334.3648137

The manufacturer's authorised representative in the EU is Springer Nature Customer Service Centre GmbH, Europaplatz 3, 69115 Heidelberg, Germany. If you have any concerns regarding our products, please contact ProductSafety@springernature.com

Printed and bound by CPI Group (UK) Ltd, Croydon, CR0 4YY
01/10/2026
02225921-0003